SAUNDERS

VETERINARY ANATOMY
COLORING BOOK

SECOND EDITION

EXPERT CONSULTANT

Baljit Singh, BVSc&AH, MVSc, PhD, FAAA

3M National Teaching Fellow
Professor and Associate Dean (Research)
Western College of Veterinary Medicine
University of Saskatchewan
Saskatoon, Saskatchewan
Canada

ELSEVIER

ELSEVIER

3251 Riverport Lane
St. Louis, Missouri 63043

SAUNDERS VETERINARY ANATOMY COLORING BOOK,
SECOND EDITION

ISBN: 978-1-4557-7684-9

Notices

International Standard Book Number: 978-1-4557-7684-9

Content Strategy Director: Penny Rudolph
Professional Content Development Manager: Jolynn Gower
Senior Content Development Specialist: Courtney Sprehe
Publishing Services Manager: Hemamalini Rajendrababu
Project Manager: Maria Bernard
Design Direction: Ryan Cook and Brian Salisbury

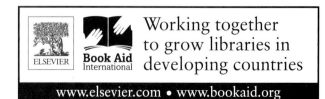

Printed in the United States of America
Last digit is the print number: 9   8   7   6

ABOUT THE COLORING BOOK

Welcome to the second edition of *Saunders Veterinary Anatomy Coloring Book!* With more than 400 illustrations for you to study and color, the coloring book is designed to help you succeed in mastering veterinary anatomy. Whether you're a student of veterinary medicine or veterinary technology, this study tool will help you memorize the anatomy you need to know and give you a fun way to review the information you have studied. The interactive exercise of adding color to the images helps you learn and retain the anatomy of the different body structures.

Saunders Veterinary Anatomy Coloring Book covers ⟲ canine, ⟲ feline, ⟲ equine, ⟲ porcine, ⟲ ruminant, ⟲ avian, and exotic—⟲ small mammals and ⟲ reptiles—anatomy, representing the range of species you need to know to be prepared to practice successfully. Each page includes a species-specific icon for easy identification of the species being covered, and the first seven sections are divided by the seven regions of the body: The Head and Ventral Neck; The Neck, Back, and Vertebral Column; The Thorax; The Abdomen; The Pelvis and Reproductive Organs; The Forelimb; and The Hindlimb.

New to this edition is Section 8: Exotics. It covers a good variety of the small mammals and reptiles you may encounter in practice.

Saunders Veterinary Anatomy Coloring Book is an ideal companion for anyone studying veterinary anatomy. Use and review this book before an examination, before class, or even before seeing your next patient.

Saunders Veterinary Anatomy Coloring Book

Each page contains a brief statement describing the body part featured and its orientation view, follow by crisp, easy-to-color illustrations. Numbered lead lines clearly identify the structures to be colored and correspond to a numbered list appearing beneath the illustration. You can create your own "color code" by using the same color to fill in the boxed number appearing on the illustration, the anatomic structure, and the corresponding numbered box on the list below the illustration. An example of a completed illustration can be found on the inside front cover.

Ackerman N, Aspinall V: *The Complete Textbook of Veterinary Nursing, ed 2,* Oxford, 2011, Butterworth -Heinemann.

Colville TP, Bassert JM: *Clinical Anatomy and Physiology for Veterinary Technicians,* ed 3, St Louis, 2015, Mosby.

Dyce KM, Sack WO, Wensing CJG: *Textbook of Veterinary Anatomy,* ed 4, St Louis, 2010, Saunders.

Evans HE, de Lahunta A: *Guide to the Dissection of the Dog,* ed 7, St Louis, 2010, Saunders.

Jepson L: *Exotic Animal Medicine: A Quick Reference Guide,* Oxford, 2009, Saunders.

Longley L: *Saunders Solutions in Veterinary Practice: Small Animal Exotic Pet Medicine,* Philadelphia, 2011, Saunders.

Mader DR: *Reptile Medicine and Surgery,* ed 2, St Louis, 2006, Saunders.

Mitchell M, Tully TN: *Manual of Exotic Pet Practice,* St. Louis, 2008, Saunders.

Quesenberry K, Carpenter JW: *Ferrets, Rabbits, and Rodents,* ed 3, St Louis, 2012, Saunders.

Silverman S, Tell L: *Radiology of Rodents, Rabbits and Ferrets,* St Louis, 2005, Saunders.

v

CONTENTS

Saunders Veterinary Anatomy Coloring Book

CONTENTS

CONTENTS

CONTENTS

CONTENTS

CONTENTS

CONTENTS

THE HEAD AND VENTRAL NECK

FIGURE 1-1

Lateral (*A*), dorsal (*B*), and ventral (*C*) views of the
canine skull to show the extents of the cranial bones

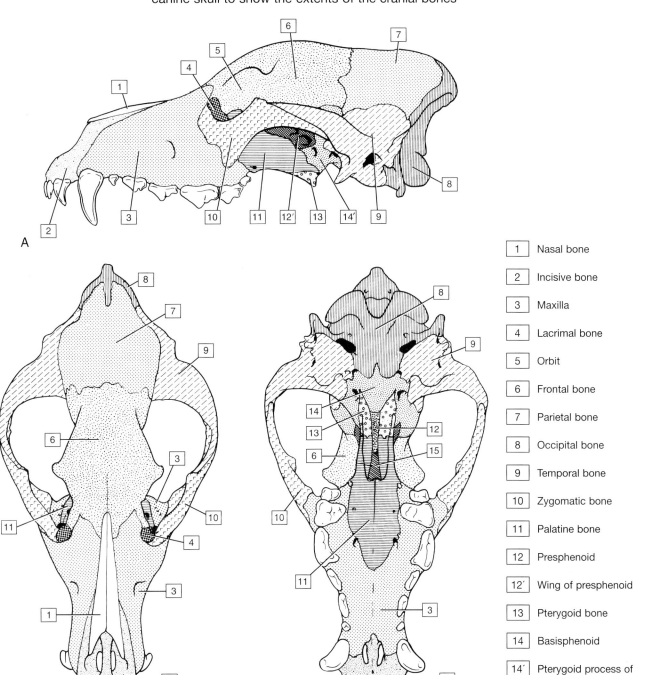

1	Nasal bone
2	Incisive bone
3	Maxilla
4	Lacrimal bone
5	Orbit
6	Frontal bone
7	Parietal bone
8	Occipital bone
9	Temporal bone
10	Zygomatic bone
11	Palatine bone
12	Presphenoid
12′	Wing of presphenoid
13	Pterygoid bone
14	Basisphenoid
14′	Pterygoid process of basisphenoid
15	Vomer

FIGURE 1-2   Dorsal View of the Canine Skull

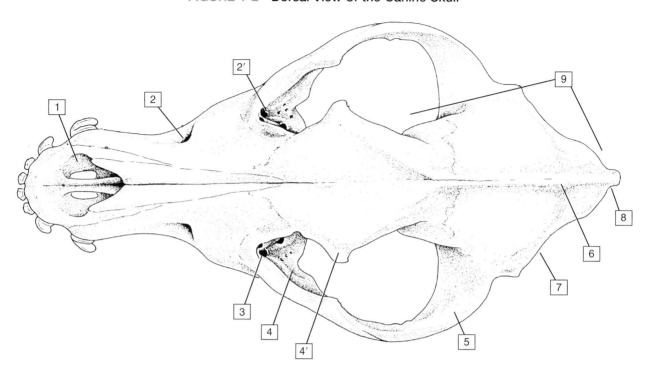

1	Nasal aperture	5	Zygomatic arch
2	Infraorbital foramen	6	External sagittal crest
2′	Maxillary foramen	7	Nuchal crest
3	Fossa for lacrimal sac	8	External occipital protuberance
4	Orbit	9	Cranium
4′	Zygomatic process of frontal bone		

Draw the outline of the occipital,
parietal, palatine, and maxilla bones.

Saunders Veterinary Anatomy Coloring Book

FIGURE 1-3 Ventral View of the Canine Skull

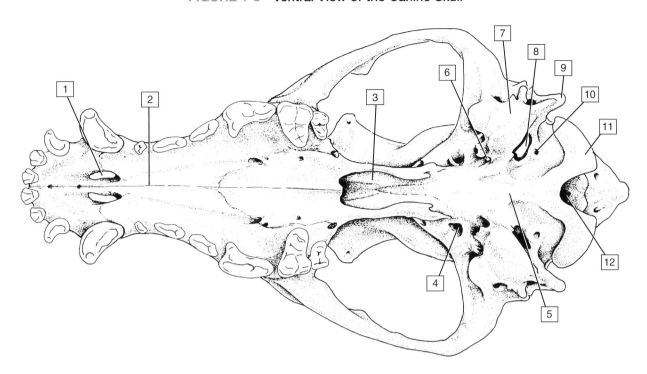

1	Palatine fissure	7	Tympanic bulla
2	Hard palate	8	Jugular foramen
3	Choanal region	9	Paracondylar process
4	Oval foramen	10	Hypoglossal canal
5	Base of cranium	11	Occipital condyle
6	Foramen lacerum	12	Foramen magnum

FIGURE 1-4   Hyoid Apparatus and Larynx Suspended
from the Temporal Region of a Canine Skull

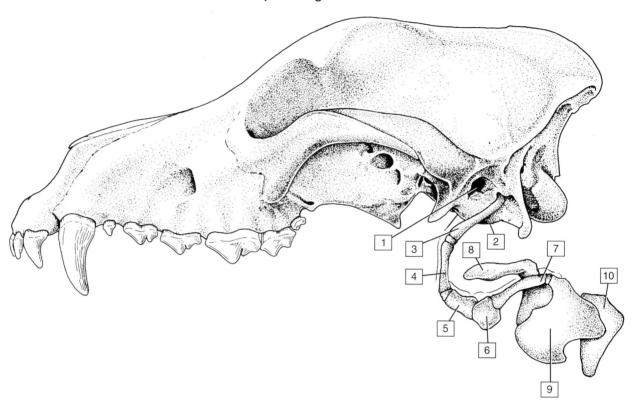

1	External acoustic meatus	6	Basihyoid
2	Tympanic bulla	7	Thyrohyoid
3	Stylohyoid	8	Epiglottic cartilage
4	Epihyoid	9	Thyroid cartilage
5	Ceratohyoid	10	Cricoid cartilage

Saunders Veterinary Anatomy Coloring Book

FIGURE 1-5   Canine Oral Cavity and Tongue

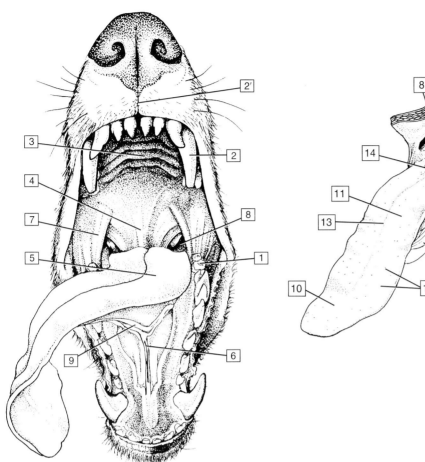
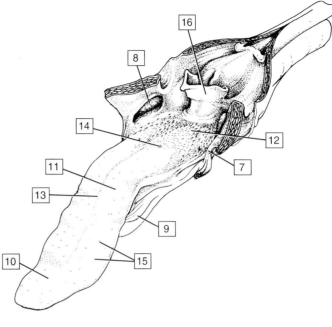

1	Vestibule	9	Frenulum
2	Canine tooth	10	Apex
2′	Philtrum	11	Body
3	Hard palate	12	Root, forming floor of oropharynx
4	Soft palate	13	Median groove
5	Tongue	14	Vallate papilla
6	Sublingual caruncle	15	Fungiform papillae
7	Palatoglossal arch	16	Epiglottis
8	Palatine tonsil		

FIGURE 1-6   Muscles of the Canine Tongue and Pharynx

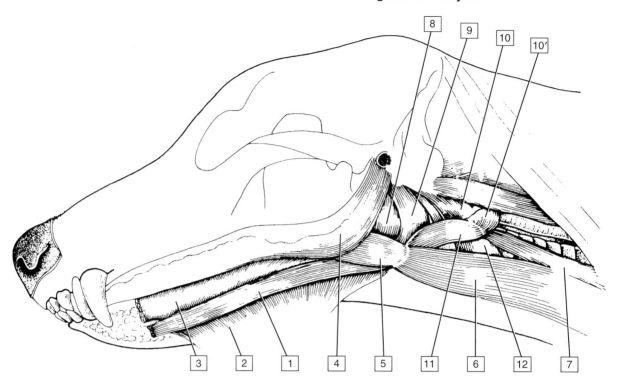

1	Geniohyoideus	8	Hyopharyngeus (two parts)
2	Mylohyoideus	9	Hyopharyngeus (two parts)
3	Genioglossus	10	Thyropharyngeus
4	Styloglossus	10′	Cricopharyngeus
5	Hyoglossus	11	Thyrohyoideus
6	Sternohyoideus	12	Cricothyroideus
7	Sternothyroideus		

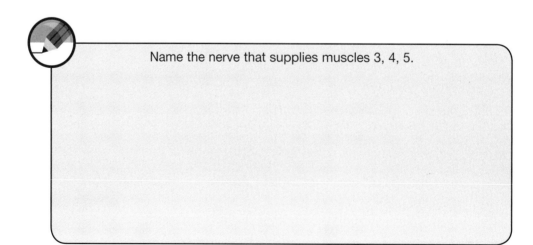

Name the nerve that supplies muscles 3, 4, 5.

Saunders Veterinary Anatomy Coloring Book

FIGURE 1-7 Canine Salivary Glands

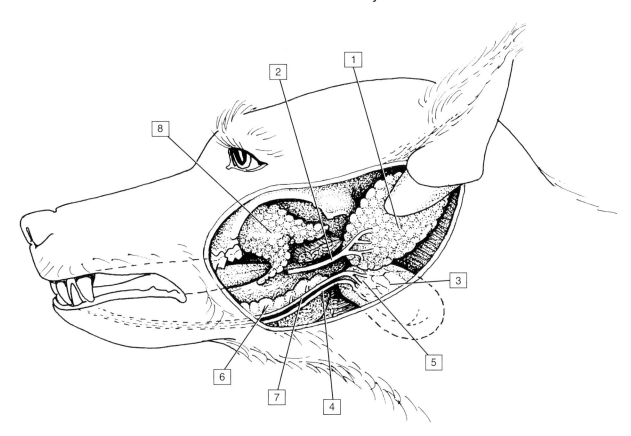

1	Parotid gland	5	Caudal part of compact sublingual gland
2	Parotid duct	6	Rostral part of compact sublingual gland
3	Mandibular gland	7	Major sublingual duct
4	Mandibular duct	8	Zygomatic gland

FIGURE 1-8

Canine simple tooth *(A)* and muscles of
mastication in lateral views *(B)* and in a section *(C)*

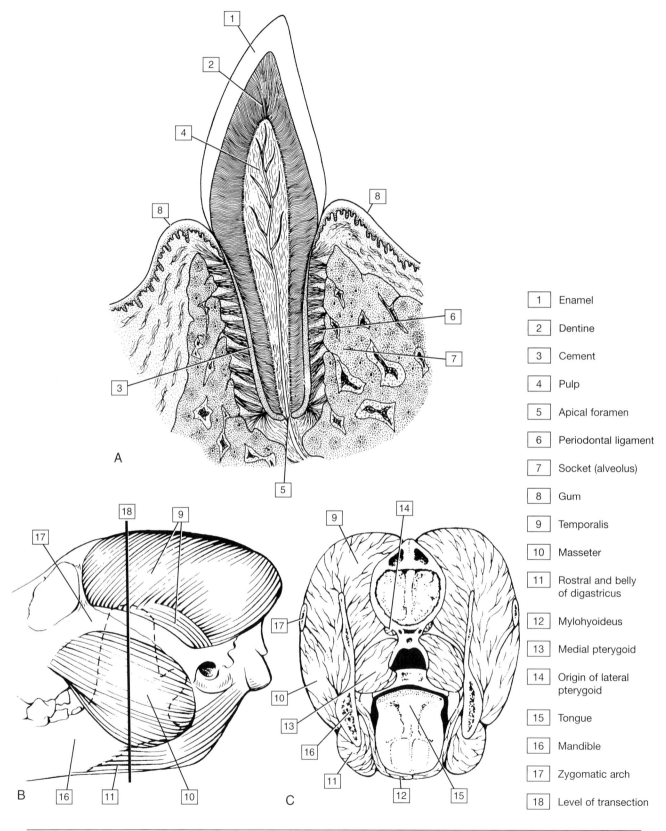

1	Enamel
2	Dentine
3	Cement
4	Pulp
5	Apical foramen
6	Periodontal ligament
7	Socket (alveolus)
8	Gum
9	Temporalis
10	Masseter
11	Rostral and belly of digastricus
12	Mylohyoideus
13	Medial pterygoid
14	Origin of lateral pterygoid
15	Tongue
16	Mandible
17	Zygomatic arch
18	Level of transection

FIGURE 1-9 Development of Canine Dental Plate and Enamel Organ

A, Development of canine dental plate, and
B, C, enamel organ. *D,* Deciduous tooth before eruption.

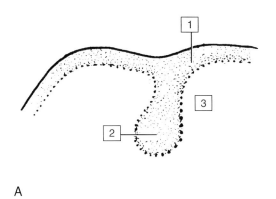

A

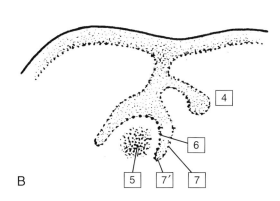

B

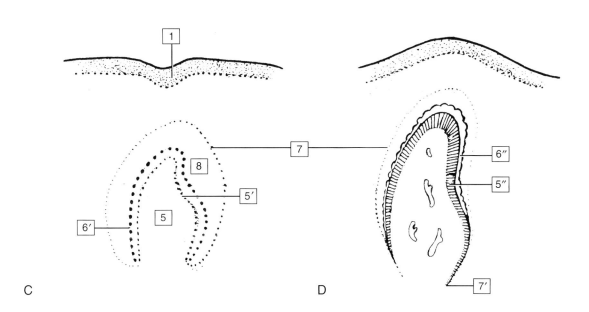

C   D

1	Epithelium of oral cavity	5	Dental papilla
2	Dental plate	5′	Odontoblasts (differentiated from the outer cell layer of the papilla)
3	Mesenchyme		
4	Bud of a permanent tooth	5″	Dentine

6	Inner dental epithelium (future ameloblasts)
6′	Ameloblasts
6″	Enamel
7	Outer dental epithelium

7′	Transition of inner and outer dental epithelia (where root formation occurs)
8	Enamel reticulum

FIGURE 1-10   Transverse Section of the Canine Larynx

Arrows on the left: action of cricoarytenoideus lateralis on arytenoid cartilage.
Arrows on the right: action of cricoarytenoideus dorsalis on arytenoid cartilage.

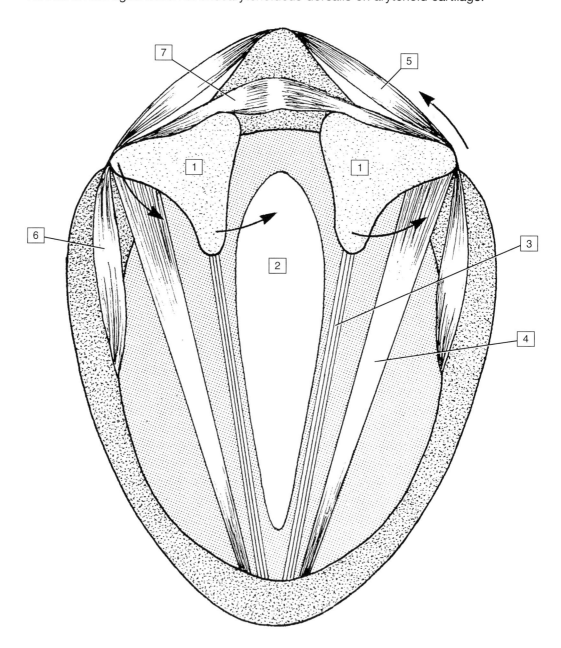

1	Location of the cricoarytenoid joint
2	Glottic cleft
3	Vocal ligament in vocal fold
4	Thyroarytenoideus

5	Cricoarytenoideus dorsalis
6	Cricoarytenoideus lateralis
7	Arytenoideus transversus

Name the nerve that supplies muscles 4, 5, 6, and 7.

FIGURE 1-11 Organization of the Canine
Brain-Pituitary-Peripheral Organ Axis

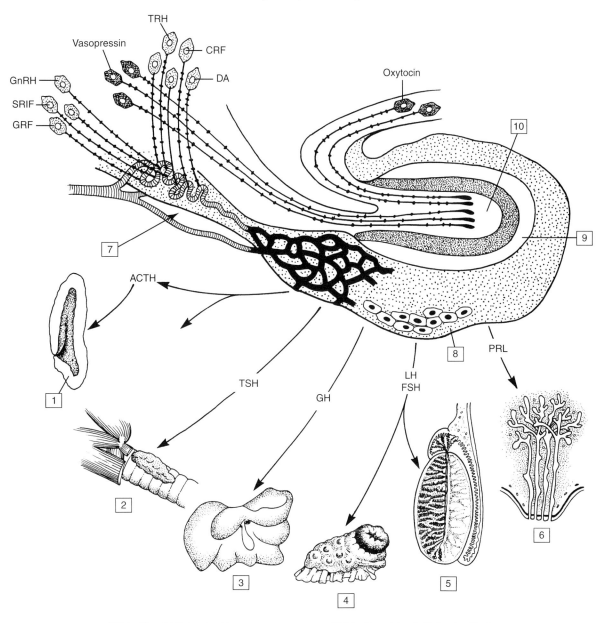

TRH = Thyroid-Releasing Hormone
CRF = Corticotropin-Releasing Factor
DA = Dopamine
GnRH = Gonadotropin-Releasing Hormone
SRIF = Somatotropin-Release Inhibiting Factor

GRF = Gonadotropin-Releasing Factor
ACTH = Adrenocorticotropic Hormone
TSH = Thyroid-Stimulating Hormone
GH = Growth Hormone
LH = Luteinizing Hormone
FSH = Follicle-Stimulating Hormone
PRL = Prolactin

1	Adrenal cortex	5	Testis	9	Intermediate lobe of pituitary
2	Thyroid	6	Mammary gland	10	Neural lobe of pituitary
3	Liver	7	Median eminence		
4	Ovary	8	Anterior lobe of pituitary		

FIGURE 1-12 Arteries of the Canine Head

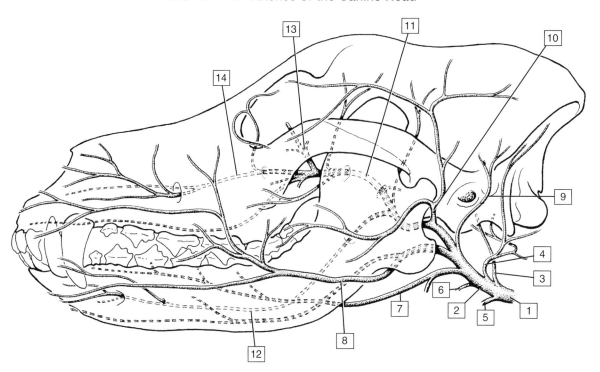

1	Common carotid a.	5	Cranial laryngeal a.	8	Facial a.	12	Inferior alveolar a.
2	External carotid a.	6	Ascending pharyngeal a.	9	Caudal auricular a.	13	External ophthalmic a.
3	Internal carotid a.	7	Lingual a.	10	Superficial temporal a.	14	Infraorbital a.
4	Occipital a.			11	Maxillary a.		

FIGURE 1-13 Canine Reflex Chain in which an Interneuron is Interposed

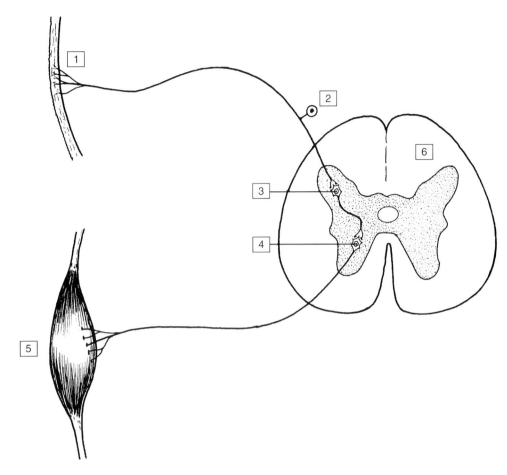

1	Skin receptor	4	Synapse at efferent neuron
2	Afferent neuron	5	Muscle
3	Synapse at interneuron	6	Spinal cord

FIGURE 1-14 The Course of Fibers within the Canine Spinal Cord

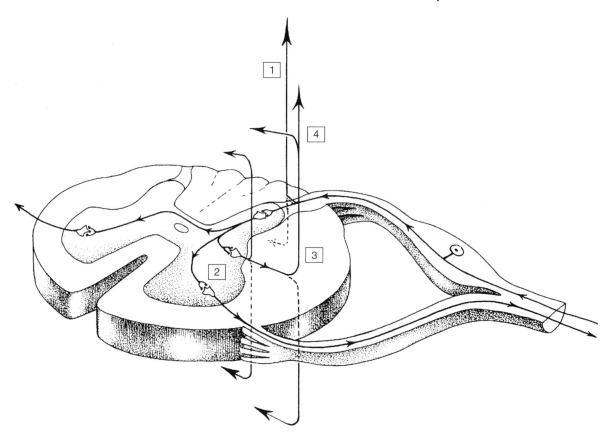

1 | Afferent fibers in the dorsal funiculus traveling toward the brain (others end on interneurons in the dorsal horn)

2 | Impulses transmitted directly to efferent neurons

3 | Impulses transmitted to other interneurons transmitting impulses caudally or cranially within the spinal cord

4 | Impulses extending to the brain

FIGURE 1-15   Dorsal View of the Canine Brain

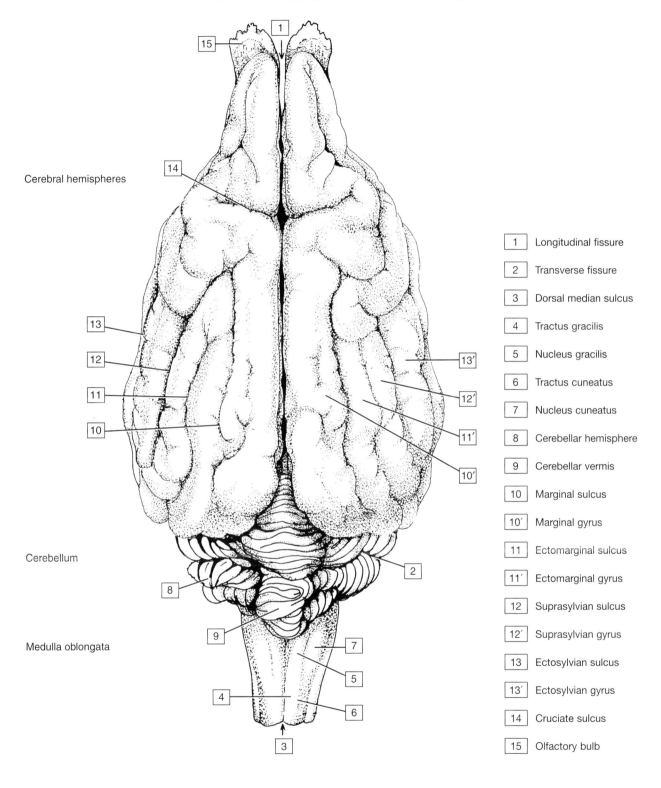

Cerebral hemispheres

Cerebellum

Medulla oblongata

1	Longitudinal fissure
2	Transverse fissure
3	Dorsal median sulcus
4	Tractus gracilis
5	Nucleus gracilis
6	Tractus cuneatus
7	Nucleus cuneatus
8	Cerebellar hemisphere
9	Cerebellar vermis
10	Marginal sulcus
10´	Marginal gyrus
11	Ectomarginal sulcus
11´	Ectomarginal gyrus
12	Suprasylvian sulcus
12´	Suprasylvian gyrus
13	Ectosylvian sulcus
13´	Ectosylvian gyrus
14	Cruciate sulcus
15	Olfactory bulb

FIGURE 1-16   Ventral View of the Canine Brain

I-XII designate the appropriate cranial nerves.

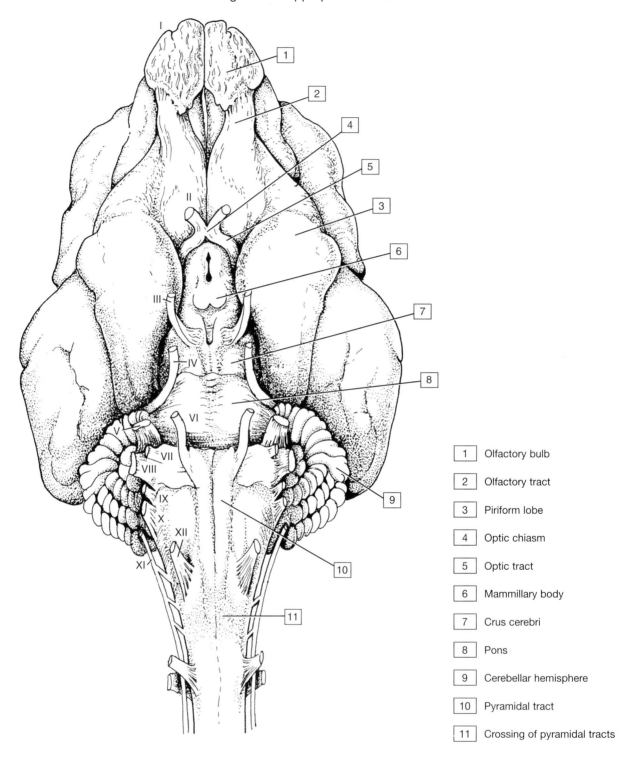

1	Olfactory bulb
2	Olfactory tract
3	Piriform lobe
4	Optic chiasm
5	Optic tract
6	Mammillary body
7	Crus cerebri
8	Pons
9	Cerebellar hemisphere
10	Pyramidal tract
11	Crossing of pyramidal tracts

FIGURE 1-17   Median Section of the Canine Brain

Part of the medial wall of the hemisphere has been removed.

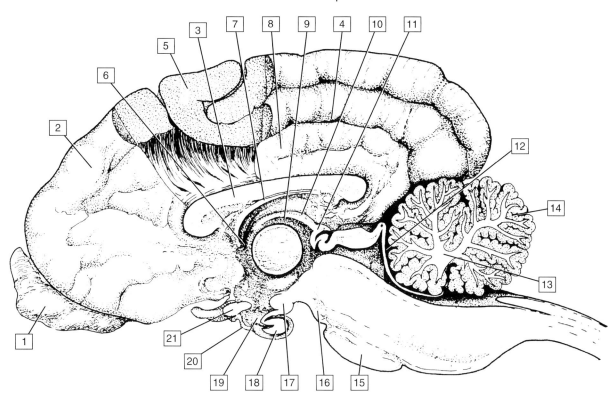

1 Olfactory bulb	12 Rostral medullary velum
2 Hemisphere	13 Corpus medullare
3 Corpus callosum	14 Cerebellar cortex
4 Splenial sulcus	15 Pons
5 Cerebral cortex	16 Crus cerebri
6 Interventricular foramen	17 Mammillary body
7 Fornix	18 Hypophysis
8 Cingulate gyrus	19 Infundibulum
9 Thalamus	20 Tuber cinereum
10 Epithalamus	21 Optic chiasm
11 Epiphysis	

FIGURE 1-18 Canine Brainstem Showing the Nuclei in an Adult Mammal

Roman numerals are used for nuclei of some cranial nerves.
A = afferent nuclei; B = efferent nuclei.

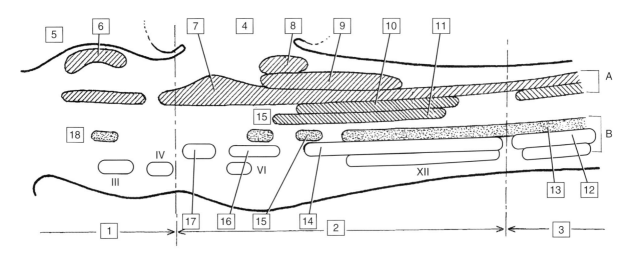

1	Mesencephalon
2	Rhombencephalon
3	Spinal cord
4	Cerebellum
5	Tectum mesencephali
6	Rostral colliculus (SSA)
7	Trigeminal nuclei (SA)
8	Cochlear nuclei (SSA)
9	Vestibular nuclei (SSA)
10	Solitary nucleus of VII, IX, X (VA)
11	Gustatory nuclei of VII, IX (SVA)
12	Motor nucleus of XI (GSE)
13	Motor nucleus of X (GVE)
14	Nucleus ambiguus of IX, X (GSE)
15	Salivatory nuclei of VII, IX (GVE)
16	Motor nucleus of VII (GSE)
17	Motor nucleus of V (GSE)
18	Parasympathetic nucleus of III (GVE)

**FIGURE 1-19   A Simplified Schema of the
Canine Visual and Pupillary Reflex Pathways**

Thick lines, special somatic visual fibers; *thin lines,*
sympathetic fibers; *broken lines,* parasympathetic fibers.

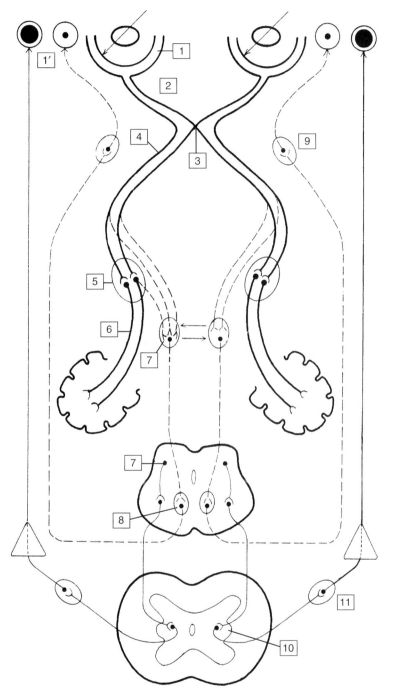

1	Retina
1′	Dilated and constricted pupils
2	Optic nerve
3	Optic chiasm
4	Optic tract
5	Lateral geniculate nucleus
6	Optic radiation
7	Rostral colliculus and pretectal nuclei
8	Oculomotor nucleus (parasympathetic part)
9	Ciliary ganglion
10	Lateral visceral efferent column
11	Cranial cervical ganglion

FIGURE 1-20   Relay Diagram of the Pyramidal (Continuous
Line) and the Extrapyramidal (Interrupted Line) Systems

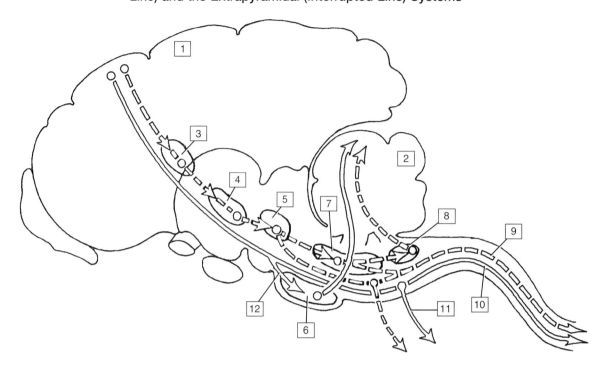

1 Motor cortex	7 Reticular formation
2 Cerebellum	8 Olivary nucleus
3 Basal nuclei	9 Rubrospinal tract
4 Substantia nigra (mesencephalon)	10 Corticospinal fibers
5 Red nucleus (mesencephalon)	11 Corticobulbar fibers
6 Pontine nuclei (metencephalon)	12 Corticopontine fibers

Saunders Veterinary Anatomy Coloring Book

FIGURE 1-21   Arteries on the Ventral Surface of the Canine Brain

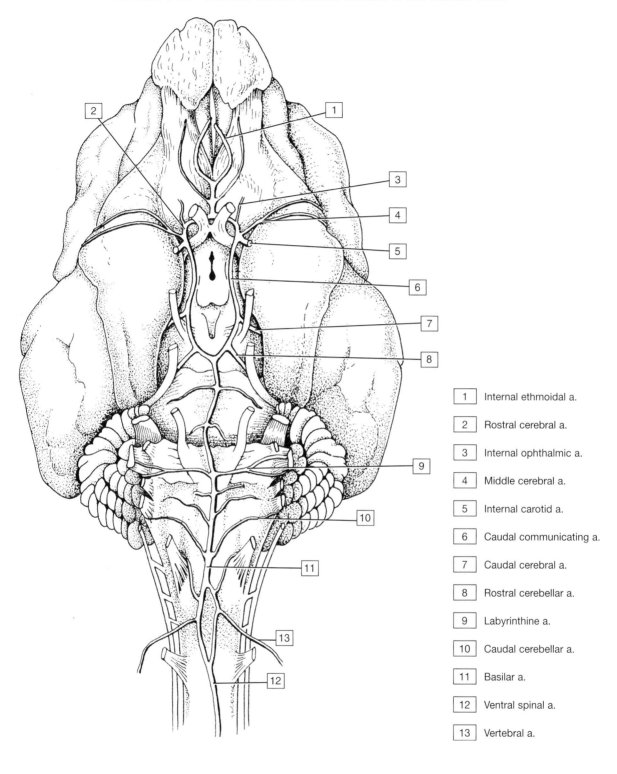

1	Internal ethmoidal a.
2	Rostral cerebral a.
3	Internal ophthalmic a.
4	Middle cerebral a.
5	Internal carotid a.
6	Caudal communicating a.
7	Caudal cerebral a.
8	Rostral cerebellar a.
9	Labyrinthine a.
10	Caudal cerebellar a.
11	Basilar a.
12	Ventral spinal a.
13	Vertebral a.

FIGURE 1-22   Distribution Pattern of the Canine Facial Nerve

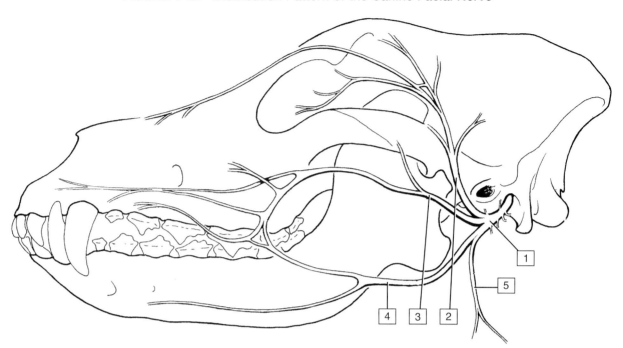

1	Facial n.	4	Ventral buccal branch
2	Auriculopalpebral n.	5	Cervical branch
3	Dorsal buccal branch		

FIGURE 1-23   Canine Eye Opened to Show the Three Tunics, which have been Drawn Thicker than they Actually are

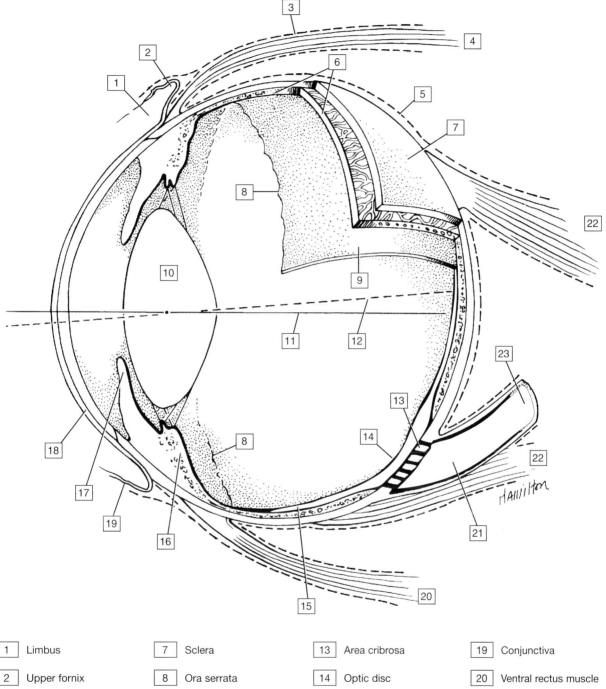

1	Limbus	7	Sclera	13	Area cribrosa	19	Conjunctiva
2	Upper fornix	8	Ora serrata	14	Optic disc	20	Ventral rectus muscle
3	Deep muscular fascia	9	Retina	15	Retina	21	Optic nerve
4	Dorsal rectus muscle	10	Lens	16	Ciliary body	22	Retractor bulbi
5	Vagina bulbi	11	Optic axis	17	Iris	23	Sheath of optic nerve
6	Choroid	12	Visual axis	18	Cornea		

FIGURE 1-24 Anterior Part of the Canine Eye in Section

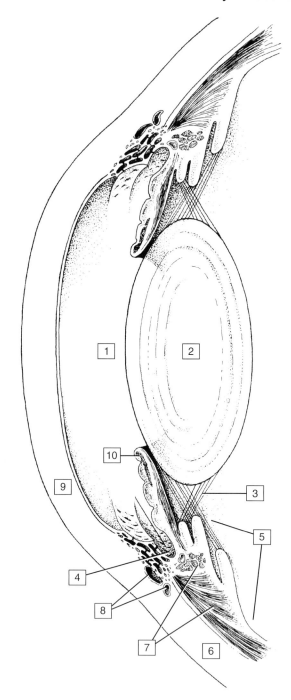

1	Anterior chamber	6	Sclera
2	Lens	7	Ciliary muscles
3	Zonular fibers	8	Venous plexus of sclera
4	Iridocorneal angle	9	Cornea
5	Ciliary body	10	Iris with the sphincter and dilator muscles shown

Saunders Veterinary Anatomy Coloring Book

FIGURE 1-25 Stumps of Canine Ocular
Muscles Viewed from Behind the Left Eyeball

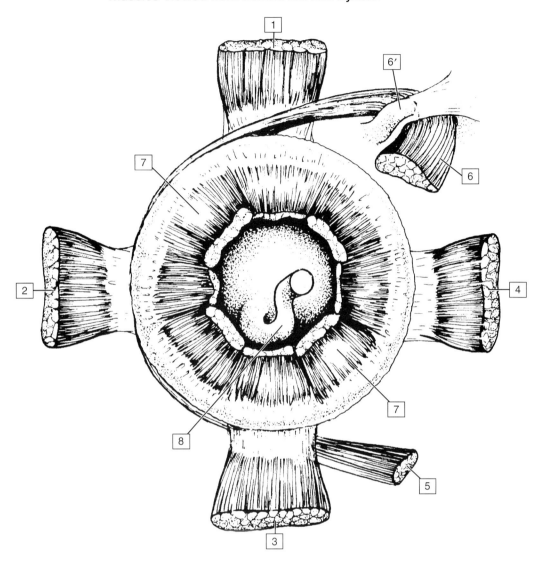

1	Dorsal rectus m.	6	Dorsal oblique m.
2	Lateral rectus m.	6′	Trochlea
3	Ventral rectus m.	7	Retractor bulbi
4	Medial rectus m.	8	Optic nerve
5	Ventral oblique m.		

FIGURE 1-26 Schema of the Right Ear, Caudal View

I: Internal ear, II: Middle ear, III: External ear

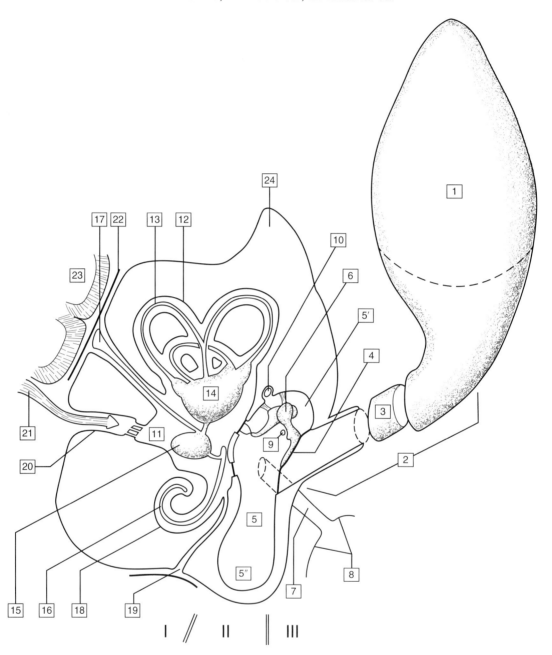

1	Auricle	6	Auditory ossicles	13	Semicircular ducts	20	Internal acoustic meatus
2	External acoustic meatus	7	Auditory tube	14	Utriculus	21	Vestibulocochlear nerve in internal acoustic meatus
3	Annular cartilage	8	Nasopharynx	15	Sacculus	22	Meninges
4	Tympanic membrane	9	Chorda tympani	16	Cochlear duct	23	Brain
5	Tympanic cavity	10	Facial nerve	17	Endolymphatic duct	24	Petrous temporal bone
5′	Epitympanic recess	11	Vestibule	18	Cochlea		
5″	Tympanic bulla	12	Semicircular canals	19	Perilymphatic duct		

FIGURE 1-27   Canine Sensory Nerve Endings of the Skin

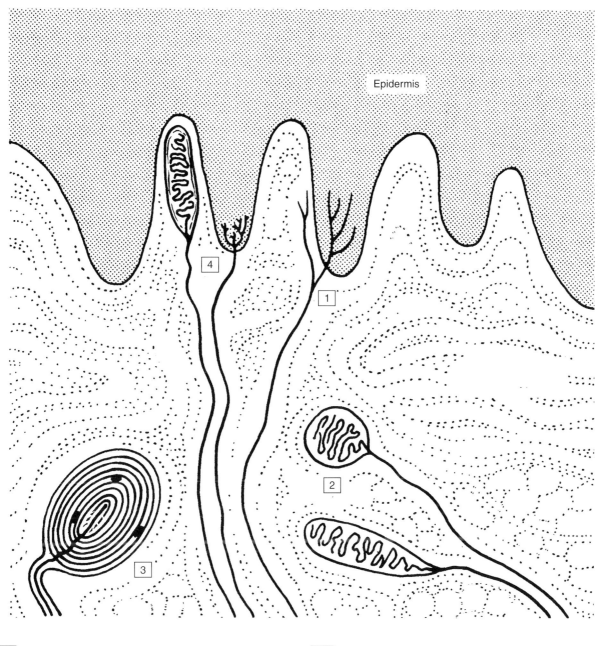

Epidermis

1	Free nerve endings (pain)	3	Lamellar corpuscles (vibration)
2	Bulbous corpuscles (heat or cold)	4	Meniscoid nerve endings (touch)

FIGURE 1-28   Canine Hair Follicle with Accessory Structures

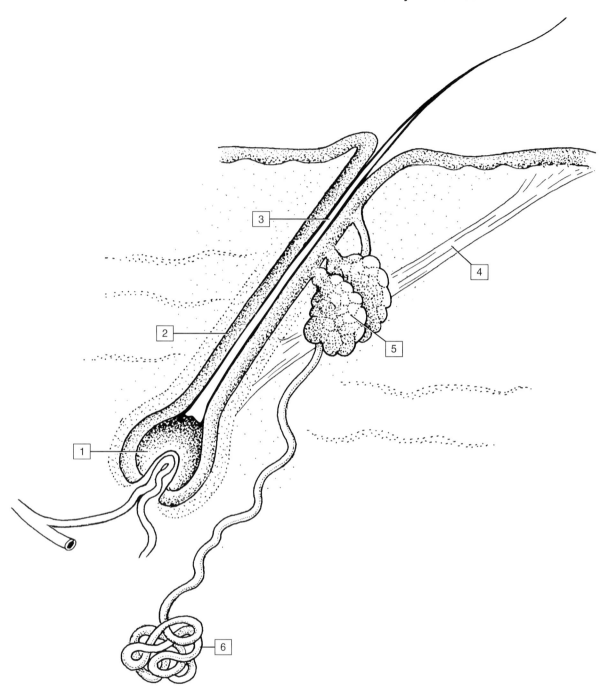

1	Bulb (hair matrix) of hair
2	Hair follicle
3	Root of hair
4	Arrector pili muscle

| 5 | Sebaceous gland |
| 6 | Sweat gland. In the adult, many glands open independently, not into hair follicles. |

FIGURE 1-29   Superficial Dissection of the Canine Head

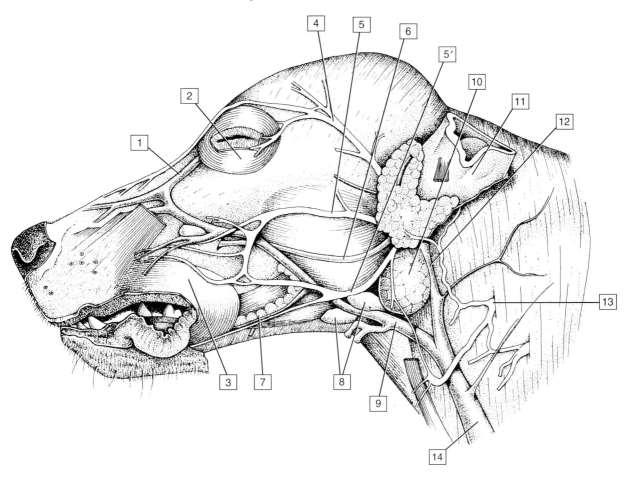

1	Angularis oculi vein	8	Mandibular lymph nodes
2	Orbicularis oculi	9	Linguofacial vein
3	Orbicularis oris	10	Mandibular gland
4	Auriculopalpebral nerve	11	Base of ear
5	Dorsal buccal branch of facial nerve	12	Maxillary vein
5′	Ventral buccal branch of facial nerve	13	Second cervical nerve
6	Parotid duct	14	External jugular vein
7	Buccal salivary glands		

FIGURE 1-30   Dissection of the Canine
Orbit and Pterygopalatine Fossa, Lateral View

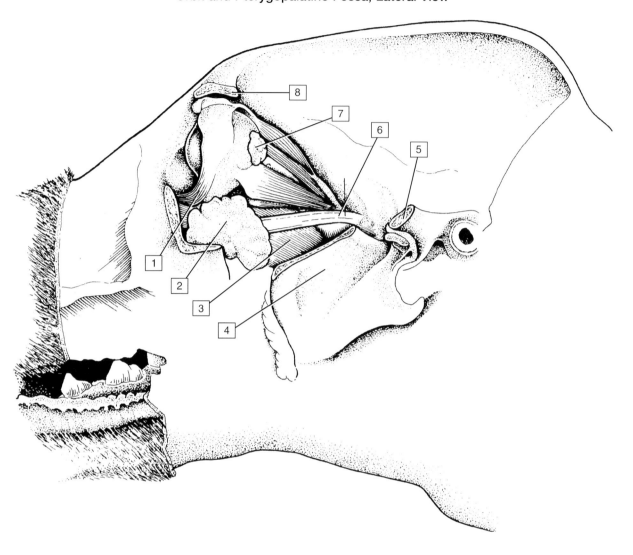

1	Ventral oblique muscle		5	Caudal stump of zygomatic arch
2	Zygomatic gland		6	Maxillary nerve
3	Medial pterygoid muscle		7	Lacrimal gland
4	Coronoid process of mandible, cut		8	Zygomatic process of frontal bone

FIGURE 1-31 The Major Arteries (*Gray*)
and Veins (*Black*) of the Canine Head

The ramus of the mandible has been removed.

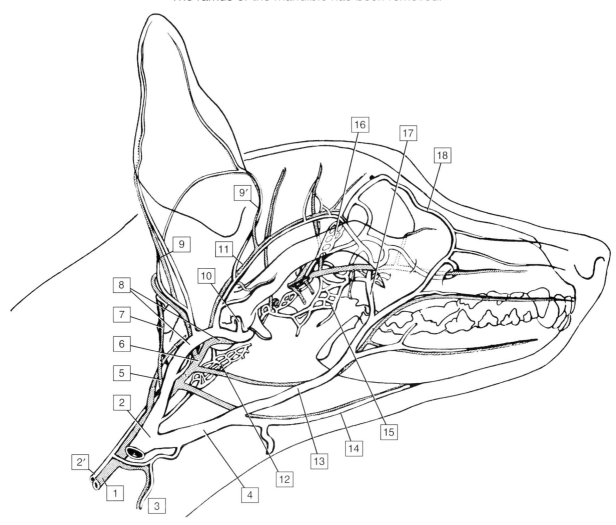

1	Common carotid	9′	Rostral auricular
2	External jugular	10	Dorsal emissary
2′	Internal jugular	11	Superficial temporal
3	Cranial thyroid	12	Ventral emissary and pharyngeal plexus
4	Linguofacial	13	Facial
5	Internal carotid	14	Lingual
6	External carotid	15	Pterygoid plexus
7	Occipital	16	Ophthalmic plexus
8	Maxillary	17	Deep facial
9	Caudal auricular	18	Angularis oculi

FIGURE 1-32   Transverse Section of the Canine
Neck at the Level of the Fifth Cervical Vertebra

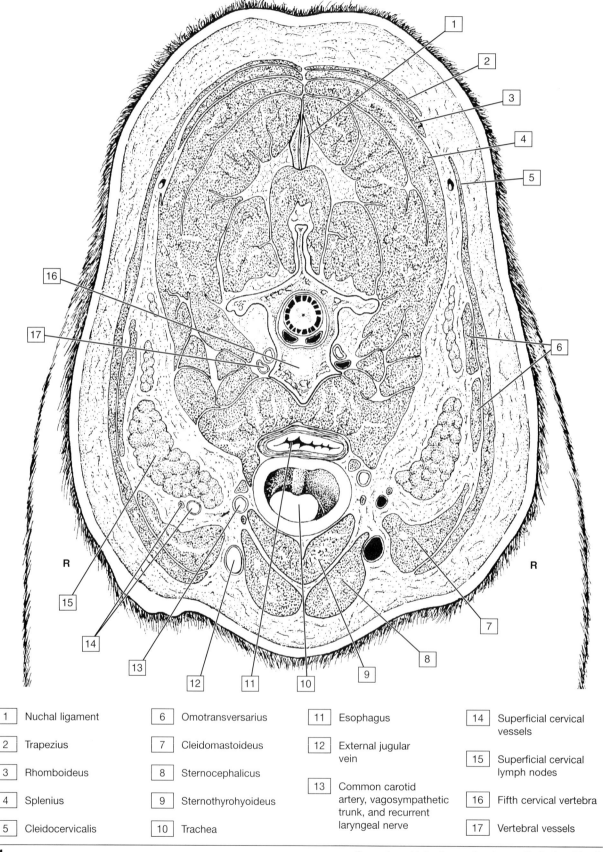

1	Nuchal ligament	6	Omotransversarius	11	Esophagus	14	Superficial cervical vessels
2	Trapezius	7	Cleidomastoideus	12	External jugular vein	15	Superficial cervical lymph nodes
3	Rhomboideus	8	Sternocephalicus	13	Common carotid artery, vagosympathetic trunk, and recurrent laryngeal nerve	16	Fifth cervical vertebra
4	Splenius	9	Sternothyrohyoideus			17	Vertebral vessels
5	Cleidocervicalis	10	Trachea				

FIGURE 1-33   Lymphatic Structures of the Canine Head and Neck

The inset shows the approximate areas of drainage of the principal nodes.

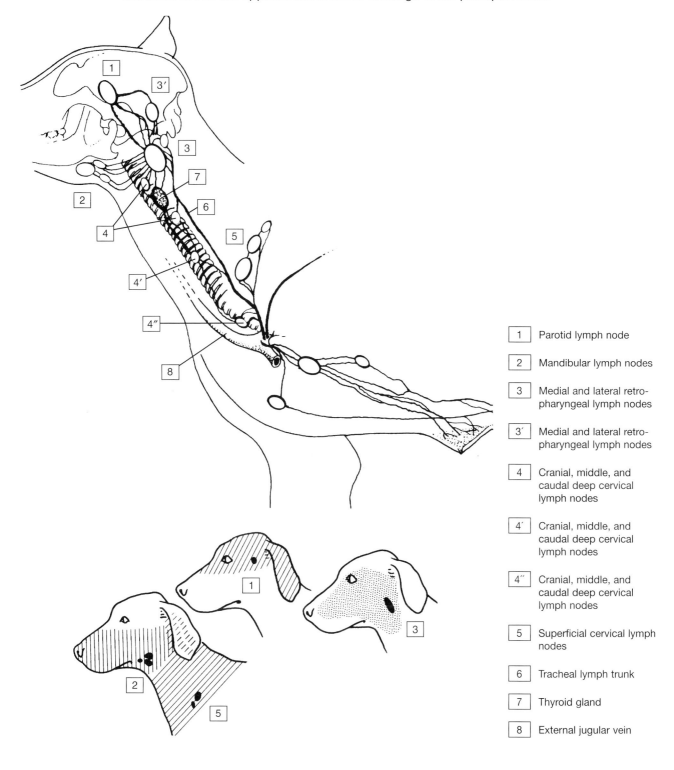

1	Parotid lymph node
2	Mandibular lymph nodes
3	Medial and lateral retro-pharyngeal lymph nodes
3′	Medial and lateral retro-pharyngeal lymph nodes
4	Cranial, middle, and caudal deep cervical lymph nodes
4′	Cranial, middle, and caudal deep cervical lymph nodes
4″	Cranial, middle, and caudal deep cervical lymph nodes
5	Superficial cervical lymph nodes
6	Tracheal lymph trunk
7	Thyroid gland
8	External jugular vein

FIGURE 1-34   Superficial Nerves of the Canine Neck, Lateral Aspect

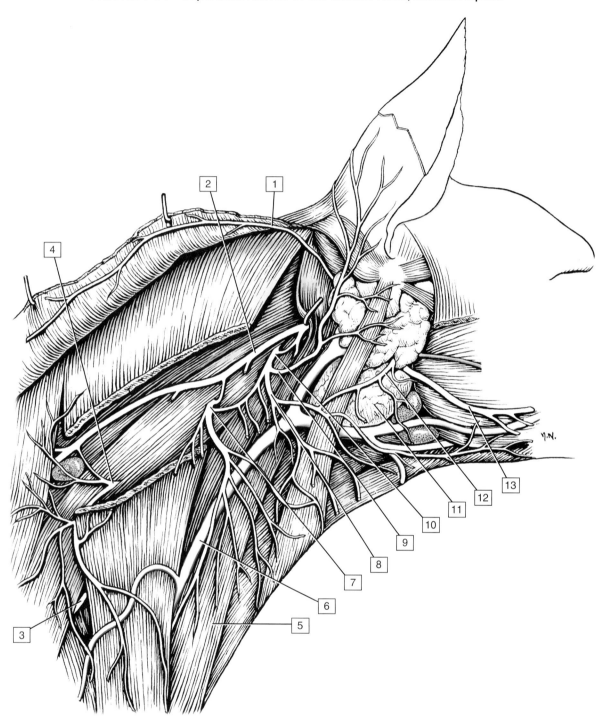

1	Caudal auricular nerve (VII)	5	Sternocephalicus	9	Great auricular nerve	13	VII, ventral buccal branch
2	Accessory nerve	6	External jugular vein	10	C2, ventral branch		
3	C5, ventral branch	7	C3, ventral branch	11	Mandibular gland		
4	C4, ventral branch	8	Transverse cervical nerve	12	VII, cervical branch		

Saunders Veterinary Anatomy Coloring Book

FIGURE 1-35   Veins of the Canine Neck, Ventral Aspect

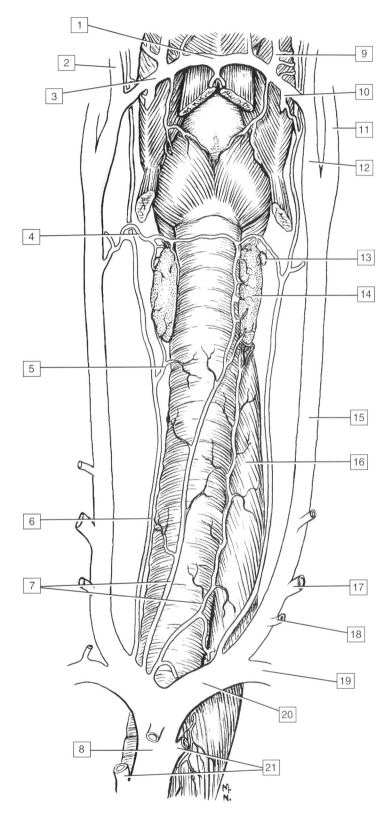

1	Hyoid venous arch
2	Facial
3	Lingual
4	Cranial thyroid
5	Middle thyroid
6	Right internal jugular
7	Caudal thyroid veins
8	Cranial vena cava
9	Lingual
10	Cranial laryngeal
11	Maxillary
12	Linguofacial
13	Parathyroid gland
14	Thyroid gland
15	External jugular
16	Esophagus
17	Superficial cervical
18	Cephalic
19	Subclavian
20	Brachiocephalic
21	Costocervical veins

FIGURE 1-36   Disarticulated Puppy Skull, Ventral View

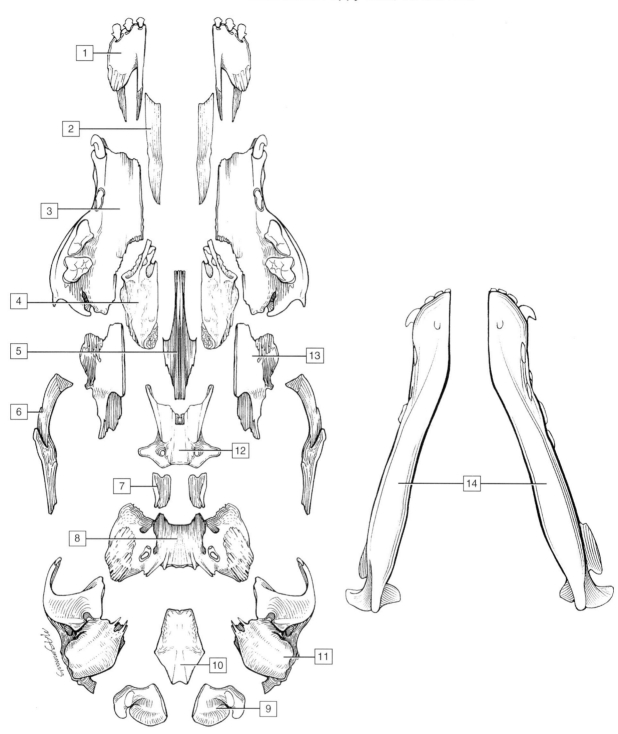

1 Incisive	5 Vomer	9 Exoccipital	12 Presphenoid
2 Nasal	6 Zygomatic	10 Basioccipital	13 Palatine
3 Maxilla	7 Pterygoid	11 Temporal	14 Mandible
4 Ethmoid	8 Basisphenoid		

FIGURE 1-37   Muscles of the Canine Pharynx and
Tongue, Left Lateral View, Left Mandible Removed

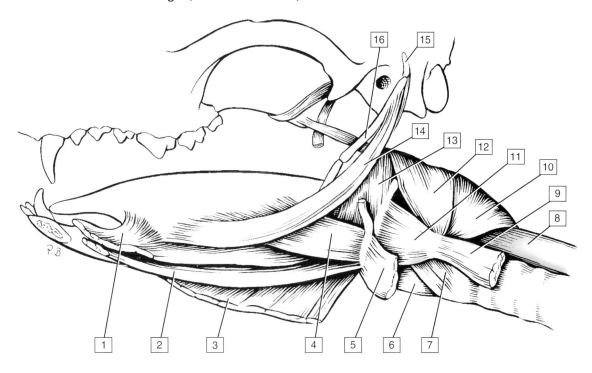

1	Genioglossus	9	Sternothyroideus
2	Geniohyoideus	10	Cricopharyngeus
3	Mylohyoideus	11	Thyrohyoideus
4	Hypoglossus	12	Thyropharyngeus
5	Sternohyoideus	13	Hyopharyngeus
6	Thyroid cartilage	14	Styloglossus
7	Cricothyroideus	15	Tympanohyoid cartilage
8	Esophagus	16	Stylohyoid bone

FIGURE 1-38 Canine Extrinsic Ocular
Muscles and their Action on the Left Eyeball

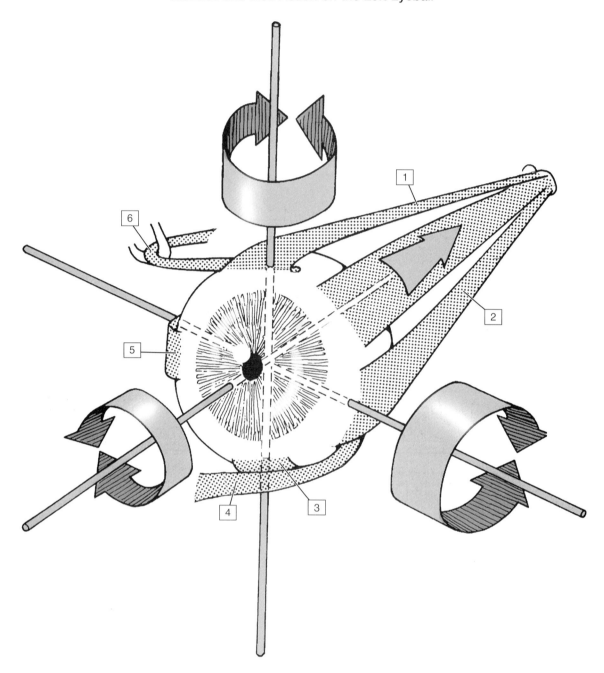

1	Dorsal rectus	4	Ventral oblique
2	Lateral rectus	5	Medial rectus
3	Ventral rectus	6	Dorsal oblique

FIGURE 1-39   Superficial Branches of
the Canine Facial and Trigeminal Nerves

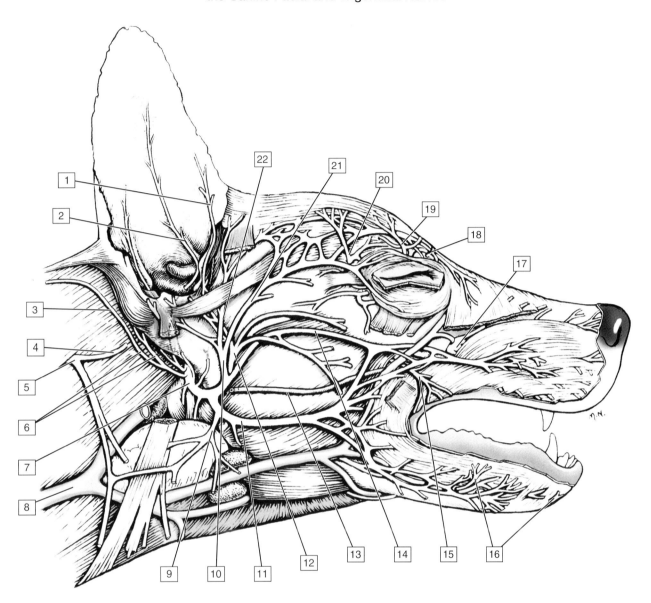

1	Rostral auricular nerve	7	Facial nerve VII	13	Parotid duct (cut)	19	Frontal nerve
2	Internal auricular branch	8	External jugular vein	14	Dorsal buccal branch	20	Zygomaticotemporal nerve
3	Caudal auricular branch to platysma	9	Cervical branch	15	Buccalis nerve	21	Palpebral nerve
4	Great auricular nerve	10	Auriculopalpebral nerve	16	Mental nerves	22	Rostral auricular nerve
5	C2, ventral branch	11	Ventral buccal branch	17	Infraorbital nerve		
6	Caudal auricular branches	12	Auriculotemporal nerve V	18	Infratrochlear nerve		

FIGURE 1-40   Branches of Canine Common Carotid Artery, Superficial Lateral View, Part of Digastricus Removed

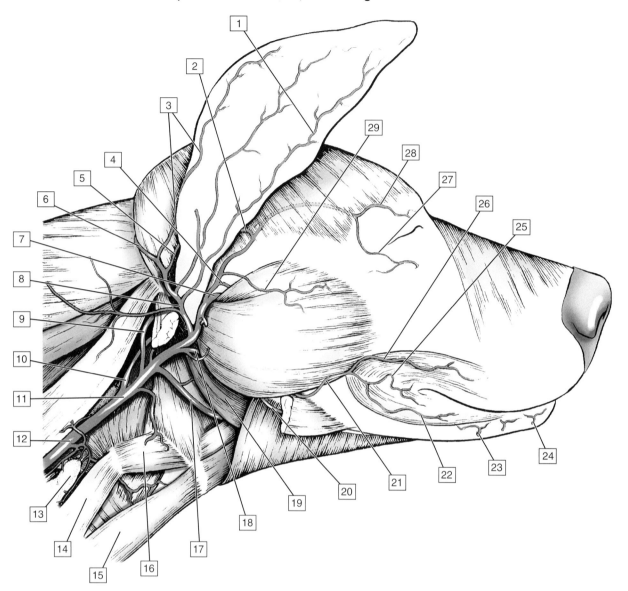

1	Lateral auricular	9	Occipital	17	Lingual	25	Angularis oris
2	Rostral auricular	10	Internal carotid	18	Facial	26	Superior labial
3	Medial auricular	11	External carotid	19	Styloglossus	27	Lateral ventral palpebral
4	Superficial temporal	12	Common carotid	20	Sublingual	28	Lateral dorsal palpebral
5	Deep auricular	13	Thyroid gland	21	Facial	29	Transverse facial
6	Occipital branch	14	Sternothyroid	22	Inferior labial		
7	Maxillary	15	Sternohyoideus	23	Caudal mental		
8	Caudal auricular	16	Thyrohyoideus	24	Rostral mental		

FIGURE 1-41 Canine Muscles, Nerves, and Salivary
Glands Medial to Right Mandible, Lateral View

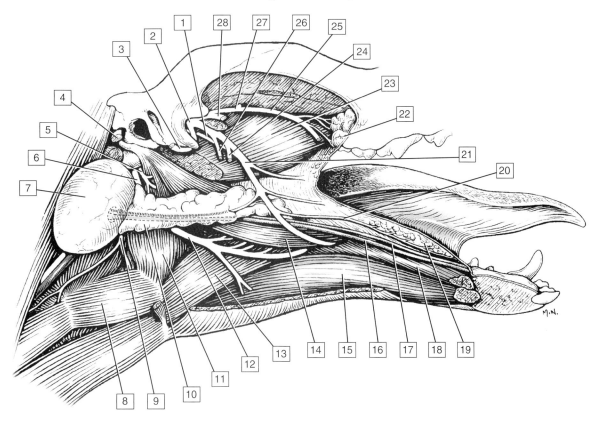

1	Chorda tympani	15	Geniohyoideus
2	Mandibular branch of V	16	Mandibular duct
3	Auriculotemporal nerve	17	Sublingual duct
4	Facial nerve	18	Genioglossus
5	Glossopharyngeal nerve	19	Polystomatic sublingual gland
6	Hypoglossal nerve	20	Sublingual nerve
7	Mandibular gland	21	Lingual nerve
8	Thyrohyoideus	22	Zygomatic gland
9	Cranial laryngeal nerve	23	Medial pterygoid
10	Monostomatic sublingual gland	24	Inferor alveolar nerve
11	Hyopharyngeus	25	Buccal nerve
12	Hypoglossal nerve	26	Mylohyoid nerve
13	Hypoglossus	27	Deep temporal branch
14	Styloglossus	28	Masseteric nerve

FIGURE 1-42   Meninges and Ventricles of the Canine Brain, Median Plane

Arrows indicate flow of cerebrospinal fluid.

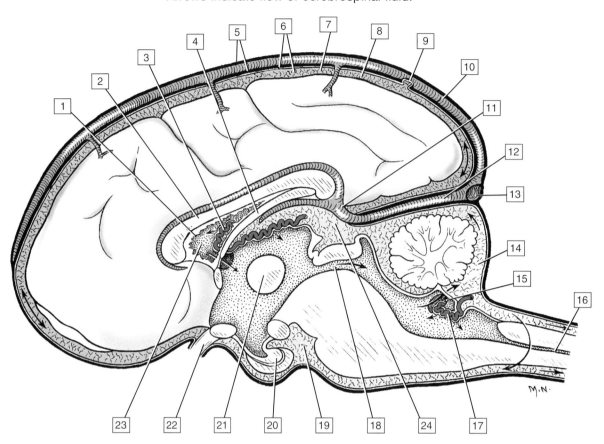

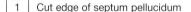

1	Cut edge of septum pellucidum		13	Transverse sinus
2	Corpus callosum		14	Cerebellomedullary cistern
3	Choroid plexus, lateral ventricle		15	Lateral aperture of fourth ventricle
4	Fornix of hippocampus		16	Central canal
5	Dura		17	Choroid plexus, fourth ventricle
6	Arachnoid membrane and trabeculae		18	Mesencephalic aqueduct
7	Subarachnoid space		19	Intercrural cistern
8	Pia		20	Neurohypophysis
9	Arachnoid villus		21	Interthalamic adhesion
10	Dorsal sagittal sinus		22	Optic nerve
11	Great cerebral vein		23	Lateral ventricle over caudate nucleus
12	Straight sinus		24	Quadrigeminal cistern

FIGURE 1-43   Ventral View of the Canine Brain, Cranial Nerves, and Brainstem

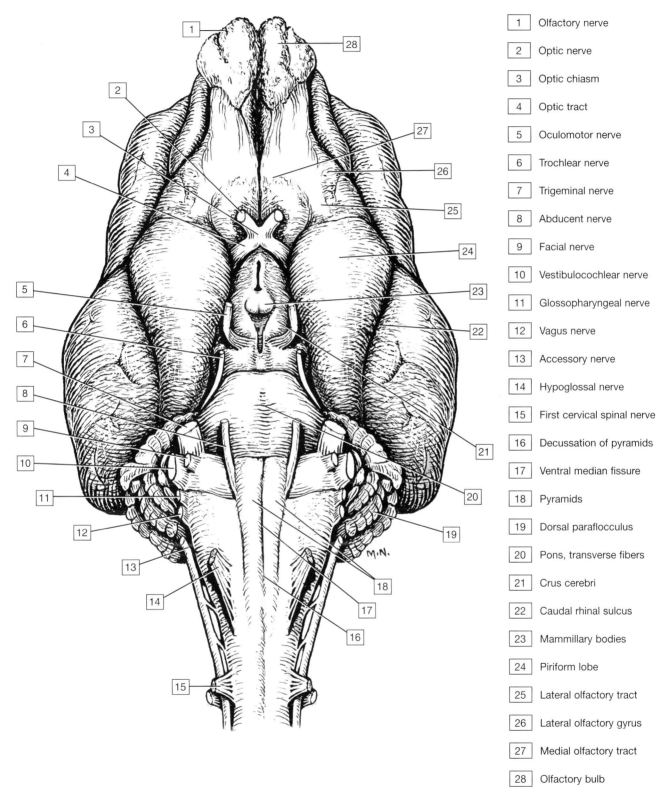

1	Olfactory nerve
2	Optic nerve
3	Optic chiasm
4	Optic tract
5	Oculomotor nerve
6	Trochlear nerve
7	Trigeminal nerve
8	Abducent nerve
9	Facial nerve
10	Vestibulocochlear nerve
11	Glossopharyngeal nerve
12	Vagus nerve
13	Accessory nerve
14	Hypoglossal nerve
15	First cervical spinal nerve
16	Decussation of pyramids
17	Ventral median fissure
18	Pyramids
19	Dorsal paraflocculus
20	Pons, transverse fibers
21	Crus cerebri
22	Caudal rhinal sulcus
23	Mammillary bodies
24	Piriform lobe
25	Lateral olfactory tract
26	Lateral olfactory gyrus
27	Medial olfactory tract
28	Olfactory bulb

FIGURE 1-44 Superficial Dissection of the Feline Head

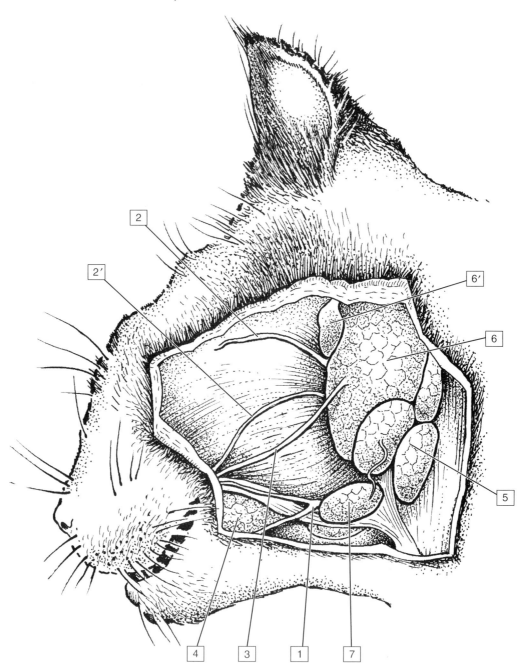

1	Facial vein	5	Mandibular gland
2	Dorsal buccal branch of facial nerve	6	Parotid gland
2′	Ventral buccal branch of facial nerve	6′	Parotid lymph node
3	Parotid duct	7	Mandibular lymph nodes
4	Buccal salivary glands		

FIGURE 1-45   Deep Dissection of the Feline
Head to Expose the Zygomatic Salivary Gland

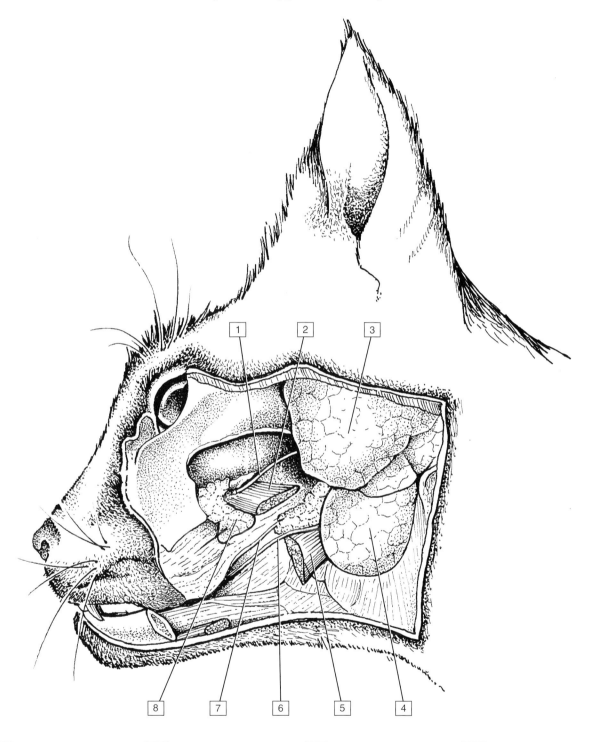

1	Parotid duct, cut	
2	Medial pterygoid muscle	
3	Parotid gland	
4	Mandibular gland	
5	Digastricus muscle	
6	Mandibular duct	
7	Sublingual duct emerging from the rostral end of the monostomatic sublingual salivary gland	
8	Zygomatic salivary gland	

FIGURE 1-46

Equine laryngeal skeleton, lateral view *(A)*, and
the intrinsic muscles of the equine larynx *(B)*.

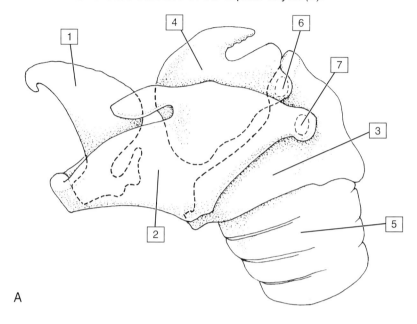

A

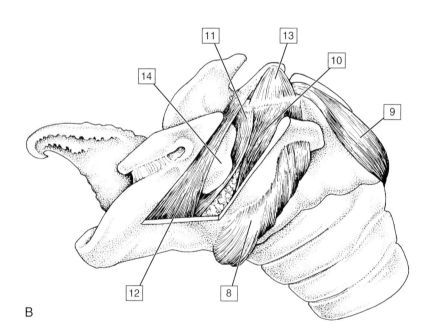

B

1	Epiglottic cartilage	5	Trachea	9	Cricoarytenoideus dorsalis	12	Ventricularis
2	Thyroid cartilage	6	Cricoarytenoid joint	10	Cricoarytenoideus lateralis	13	Arytenoideus transversus
3	Cricoid cartilage	7	Cricothyroid joint	11	Vocalis	14	Laryngeal ventricle
4	Arytenoid cartilage	8	Cricothyroideus				

Saunders Veterinary Anatomy Coloring Book

FIGURE 1-47   Anterior Half of the Left Equine Eye, Viewed from Behind

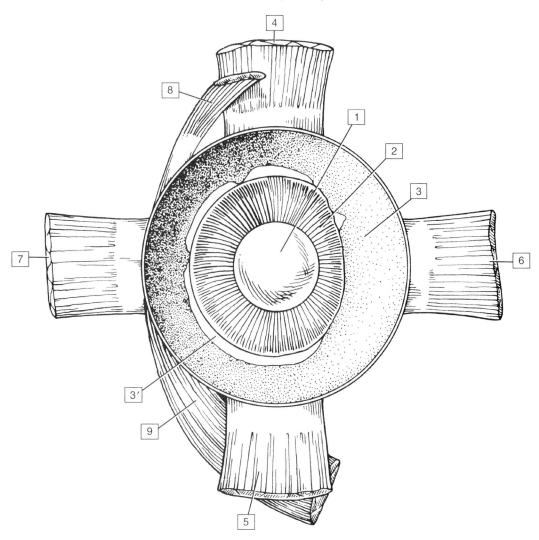

1	Lens	5	Ventral muscle
2	Ciliary body	6	Medial muscle
3	Choroid covered by pigmented outer layer of retina	7	Lateral rectus muscle
3′	Remnants of inner nervous layer of retina, which has been removed	8	Dorsal oblique muscle
		9	Ventral oblique muscle
4	Dorsal muscle		

FIGURE 1-48 Lateral View of the Equine Skull

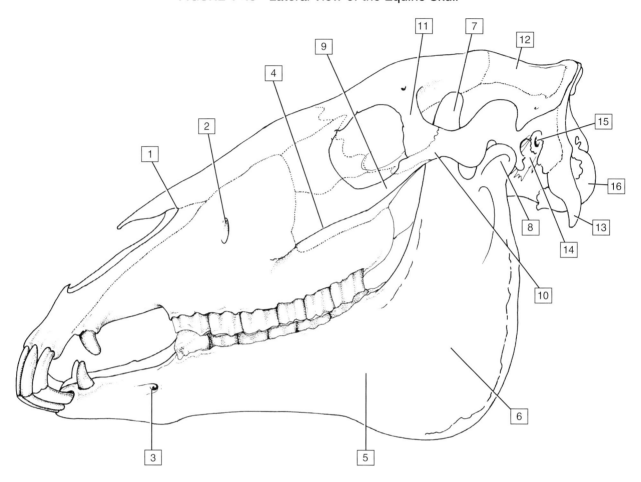

1	Nasoincisive notch		9	Temporal process of zygomatic bone
2	Infraorbital foramen		10	Zygomatic process of temporal bone
3	Mental foramen		11	Zygomatic process of frontal bone
4	Facial crest		12	External sagittal crest
5	Body of mandible		13	Paracondylar process
6	Ramus of mandible		14	Styloid process
7	Coronoid process		15	External acoustic meatus
8	Condylar process		16	Occipital condyle

FIGURE 1-49   Projection of the Brain and Frontal and
Maxillary Sinuses on the Dorsal Surface of the Equine Skull

The sinuses are filled with casting material. The frontal sinus
extends caudally over the rostal part of the brain and rostrally
beyond the level of the orbit. The circle indicates the center of the
brain and the location where a horse may be shot.

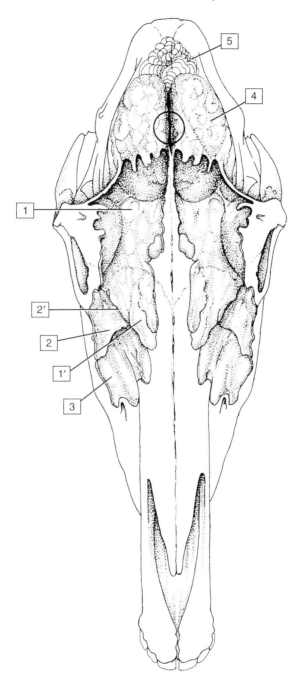

1	Conchofrontal sinus, frontal part	2	Caudal maxillary sinus	3	Rostral maxillary sinus	5	Cerebellum
1′	Conchofrontal sinus, dorsal conchal part	2′	Position of frontomaxillary opening	4	Cerebrum		

FIGURE 1-50   Structure of a Lower Equine Incisor

A, In situ, sectioned longitudinally; the clinical crown is short in relation to the embedded part of the tooth. *B,* Caudal view; the junction between the clinical crown and the rest of the tooth is not marked. *C,* As a result of wear, the occlusal surface changes; the cup gets smaller and disappears, leaving, for a time, the enamel spot: the dental star appears and changes from a line to a large round spot. *D,* These are sawn sections of a young tooth for comparison. *E,* Longitudinal section of incisor, showing the relationship between the infundibulum and dental cavity; the latter is rostral.

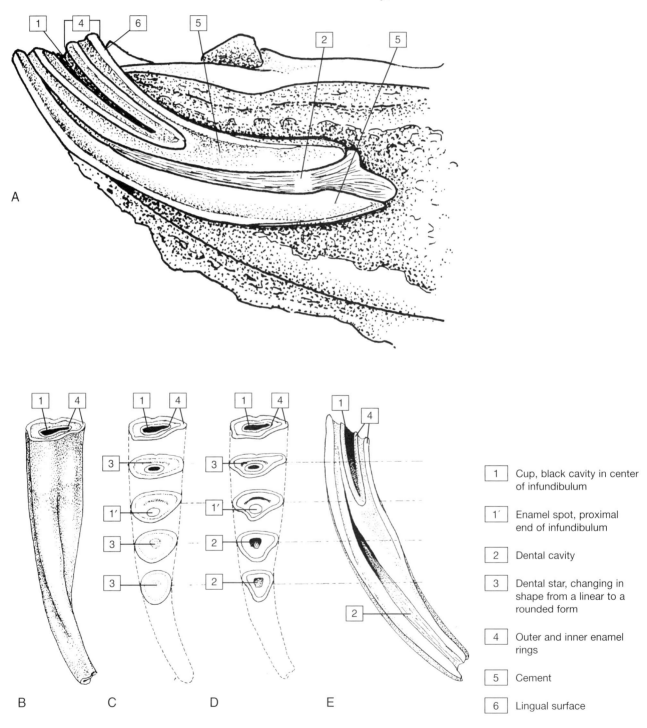

1	Cup, black cavity in center of infundibulum
1′	Enamel spot, proximal end of infundibulum
2	Dental cavity
3	Dental star, changing in shape from a linear to a rounded form
4	Outer and inner enamel rings
5	Cement
6	Lingual surface

Saunders Veterinary Anatomy Coloring Book

FIGURE 1-51 Equine Deep Masticatory Muscles and Right Digastricus

A, The deep masticatory muscles of the left side have been
exposed by removal of the left mandibular ramus (*stippled*).
B, Medial view of the right digastricus and some related structures.

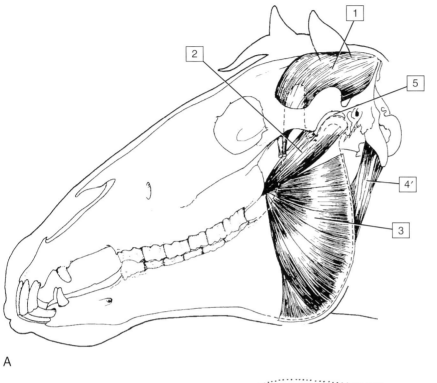

A

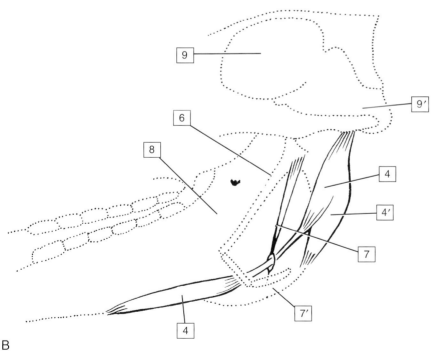

B

1	Temporalis
2	Pterygoideus lateralis
3	Lateral surface of pterygoideus medialis
4	Digastricus
4′	Occipitomandibularis
5	Left temporomandibular joint
6	Stylohyoid
7	Stylohyoideus
7′	Insertion of 7 on thyrohyoid
8	Medial surface of right mandible and mandibular foramen
9	Cranial cavity
9′	Foramen magnum

FIGURE 1-52   Muscles of the Equine
Pharynx, Soft Palate, and Hyoid Apparatus

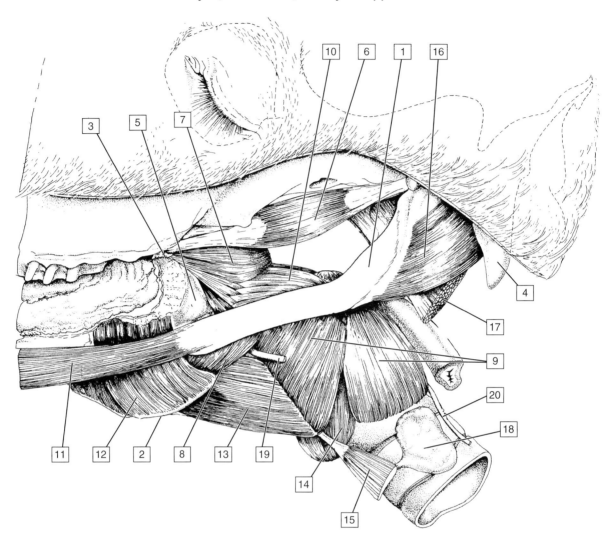

1	Stylohyoid	11	Styloglossus
2	Thyrohyoid	12	Hyoglossus
3	Hamulus of pterygoid bone	13	Thyrohyoideus
4	Paracondylar process	14	Cricothyroideus
5	Buccopharyngeal fascia	15	Sternothyroideus
6	Tensor veli palatine	16	Occipitohyoideus
7	Rostral pharyngeal constrictor	17	Longus capitis (stump)
8	Middle pharyngeal constrictor	18	Thyroid gland
9	Caudal pharyngeal constrictor (thyro- and cricopharyngeus)	19	Cranial laryngeal nerve
10	Stylopharyngeus caudalis	20	Caudal (recurrent) laryngeal nerve

FIGURE 1-53   Dissection of the Equine Orbit

The zygomatic arch and periorbita have been removed.

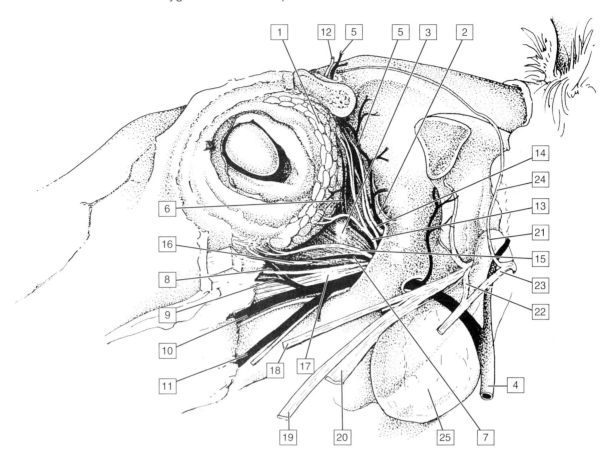

1	Lacrimal gland	14	Trochlear n.
2	Periorbita	15	Zygomatic n.
3	Lateral rectus	16	Oculomotor n.
4	Maxillary a.	17	Rostral branches of maxillary n.
5	Supraorbital a.	18	Buccal n.
6	Lacrimal a.	19	Lingual n.
7	Muscular branch of external ophthalmic a.	20	Inferior alveolar n.
8	Malar a.	21	Masticatory n.
9	Infraorbital a.	22	Auriculotemporal n.
10	Major palatine a.	23	Facial n.
11	Buccal a.	24	Auriculopalpebral n.
12	Supraorbital n.	25	Guttural pouch
13	Lacrimal n.		

FIGURE 1-54   Left Auditory Ossicles, Craniomedial View

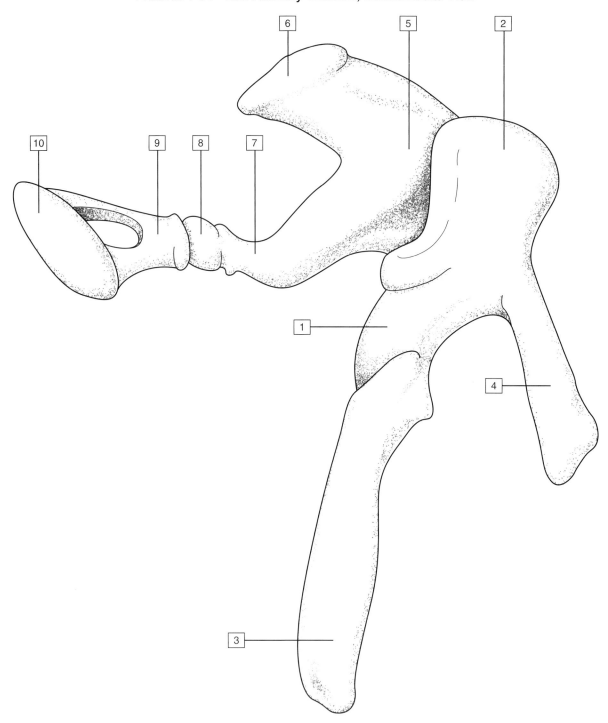

1	Malleus	4	Rostral process	7	Long crus	10	Base (footplate) of stapes
2	Head of malleus	5	Incus	8	Os lenticulare		
3	Handle of malleus	6	Short crus	9	Head of stapes		

FIGURE 1-55 Transection of the Equine Neck
at the Level of the Fourth Cervical Vertebra

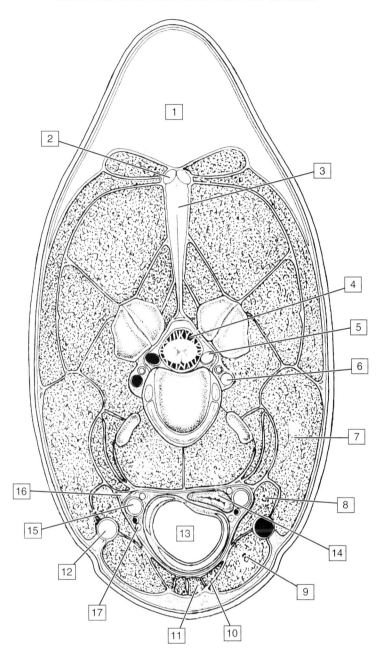

1 Crest	5 Internal vertebral venous plexus	9 Sternocephalicus	14 Esophagus
2 Funicular part of nuchal ligament	6 Vertebral artery and vein	10 Sternothyroideus	15 Common carotid artery
3 Laminar part of nuchal ligament	7 Brachiocephalicus	11 Sternohyoideus	16 Vagosympathetic trunk
4 Subarachnoid space	8 Omohyoideus	12 External jugular vein	17 Recurrent laryngeal nerve
		13 Trachea	

FIGURE 1-56   Principal Arteries of the Equine Head

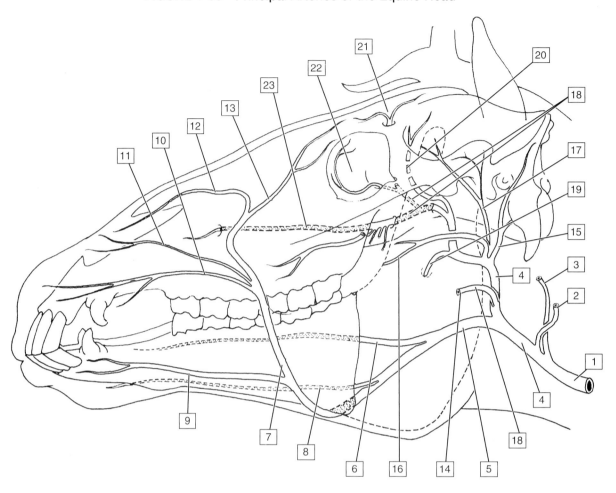

1	Common carotid a.		13	Angularis oculi a.
2	Occipital a.		14	Masseteric a.
3	Internal carotid a.		15	Caudal auricular a.
4	External carotid a.		16	Transverse facial a., displaced ventrally for clarity
5	Linguofacial a.		17	Superficial temporal a.
6	Lingual a.		18	Maxillary a.
7	Facial a.		19	Inferior alveolar a.
8	Sublingual a.		20	Caudal deep temporal a.
9	Inferior labial a.		21	Supraorbital a.
10	Superior labial a.		22	Malar a.
11	Lateral nasal a.		23	Infraorbital a.
12	Dorsal nasal a.			

FIGURE 1-57   Bovine Skull with Mandible

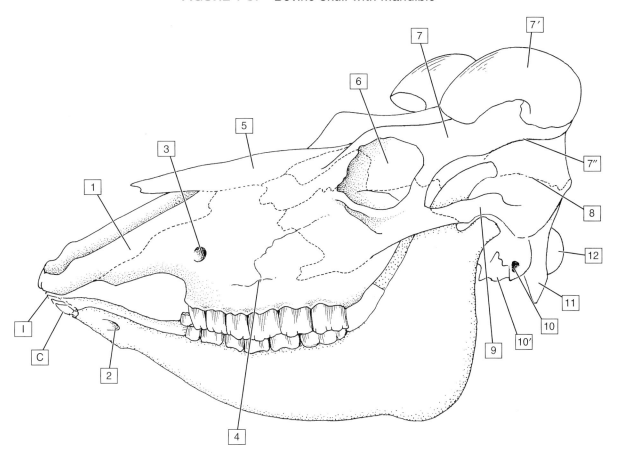

1	Incisive bone		7″	Temporal line
2	Mental foramen		8	Temporal fossa
3	Infraorbital foramen		9	Zygomatic arch
4	Facial tuberosity		10	External acoustic meatus
5	Nasal bone		10′	Tympanic bulla
6	Orbit		11	Paracondylar process
7	Frontal bone		12	Occipital condyle
7′	Horn surrounding cornual process of frontal bone			

I, Incisors; C, Canine tooth

FIGURE 1-58   Transverse Section of the Bovine Neck

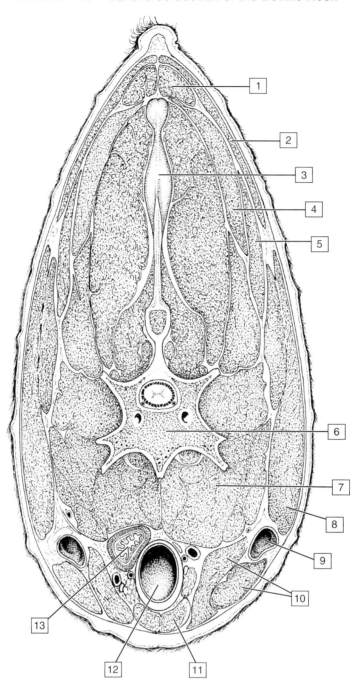

1	Rhomboideus	6	Vertebra	10	Sternocephalicus, mandibular, and mastoid parts
2	Trapezius	7	Longus colli	11	Combined sternohyoideus and sternothyroideus
3	Nuchal ligament	8	Brachiocephalicus	
4	Splenius	9	External jugular vein in jugular groove	12	Trachea
5	Omotransversarius			13	Esophagus (ventral to it, nerves, blood vessels, and thymus)

FIGURE 1-59   Right Bovine Eye Cut Along Orbital Axis, Rostromedial Surface

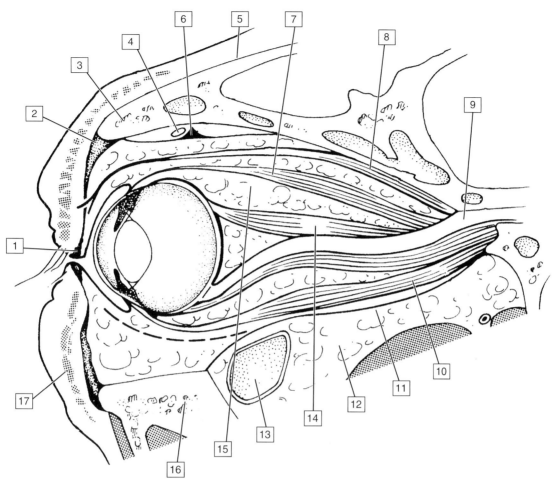

1	Tarsus	10	Ventral rectus muscle
2	Orbital septum	11	Periorbita
3	Orbital margin	12	Extraorbital fat
4	Dorsal oblique muscle	13	Lacrimal bulla, a caudal recess of the maxillary sinus
5	Periosteum of face	14	Retractor bulbi
6	Trochlea	15	Intraperiorbital fat
7	Dorsal rectus muscle	16	Zygomatic arch
8	Levator palpebrae superioris	17	Orbicularis
9	Optic nerve in optic foramen		

FIGURE 1-60 Connections of the Pharynx and
Larynx with the Base of the Bovine Skull and the Tongue

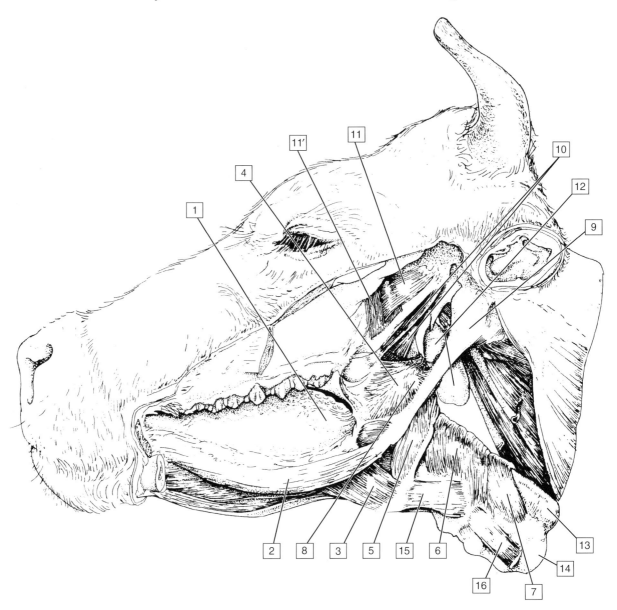

1 Root of tongue	7 Caudal pharyngeal constrictor (cricopharyngeus muscle)	12 Medial retropharyngeal lymph node
2 Styloglossus	8 Stylopharyngeus caudalis	13 Esophagus
3 Hyoglossus	9 Stylohyoid	14 Trachea
4 Rostral pharyngeal constrictor	10 Tensor and levator veli palatine	15 Thyrohyoideus
5 Middle pharyngeal constrictor	11 Pterygoideus lateralis	16 Sternothyroideus
6 Caudal pharyngeal constrictor (thyropharyngeus muscle)	11´ Remnants of pterygoideus medialis	

FIGURE 1-61   Branching of the Bovine Left Common Carotid Artery

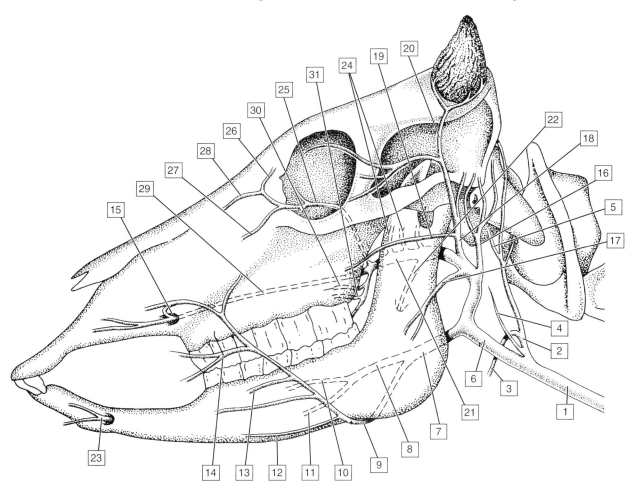

1	Common carotid a.	9	Facial a.	17	Masseteric branch	25	Malar a.
2	Occipital a.	10	Deep lingual a.	18	Superficial temporal a.	26	Angular a. of the eye
3	Ascending palatine a.	11	Sublingual a.	19	Transverse facial a.	27	Caudal lateral nasal a.
4	Remnant of internal carotid a.	12	Submental a.	20	Cornual a.	28	Dorsal nasal a.
5	Medial meningeal a.	13	Inferior labial a.	21	Maxillary a.	29	Infraorbital a.
6	External carotid a.	14	Superior labial a.	22	Inferior alveolar a.	30	Sphenopalatine a.
7	Linguofacial trunk	15	Infraorbital foramen	23	Mental a.	31	Major and minor palatine a.
8	Lingual a.	16	Caudal auricular a.	24	Rostral and caudal branches to rete mirabile		

FIGURE 1-62   Porcine Head, Superficial Dissection

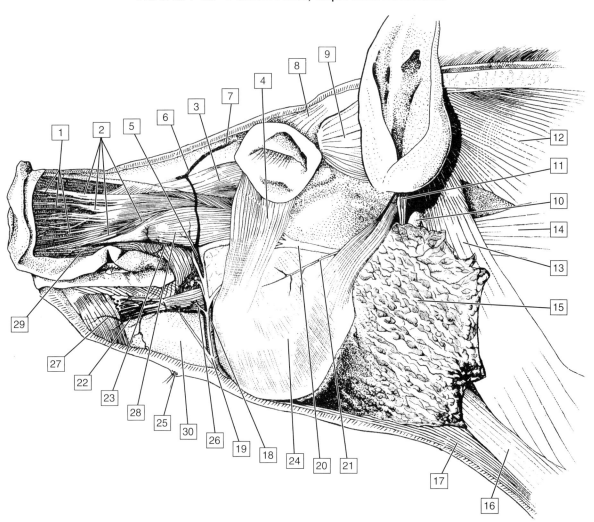

1	Cut fasciculi of levator nasolabialis	9	Frontoscutularis	17	Sternohyoideus	25	Mental hairs and gland
2	Caninus	10	Lateral retropharyngeal lymph node	18	Parotid duct	26	Depressor labii inferioris
3	Levator labii superioris	11	Parotidoauricularis	19, 20	Ventral and dorsal buccal branches of facial nerve	27	Mentalis
4	Malaris	12	Trapezius	21	Transverse facial nerve	28	Depressor labii superioris
5	Facial vein	13	Cleido-occipitalis	22	Inferior labial vein	29	Orbicularis oris
6	Dorsal nasal vein	14	Omotransversarius	23	Superior labial vein	30	Mandible
7	Frontal vein	15	Parotid gland	24	Masseter		
8	Levator anguli oculi	16	Sternocephalicus				

FIGURE 1-63   Paramedian Section of the Porcine Skull

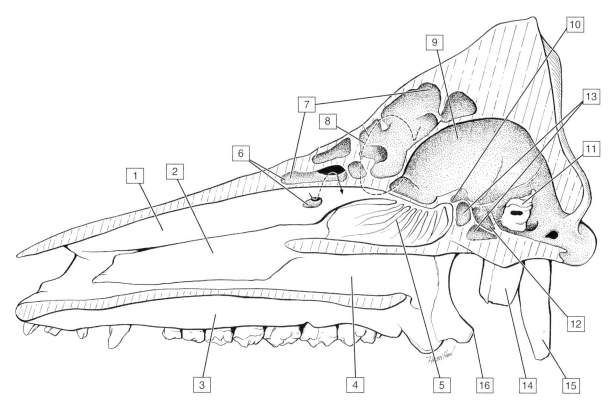

1	Dorsal turbinate bone, fenestrated at 6 to show conchal sinus
2	Ventral turbinate bone
3	Hard palate
4	Choana
5	Ethmoturbinates in fundus of nasal cavity
6	Conchal sinus
7	Portion of frontal sinus exposed by paramedian saw cut
8	Position of orbit
9	Cranial cavity
10	Optic canal
11	Petrous temporal bone
12	Fossa for hypophysis
13	Sphenoid sinus
14	Tympanic bulla
15	Paracondylar process
16	Hamulus of pterygoid bone

FIGURE 1-64   Median Section of the Head of a 4-Week-Old Pig

The nasal septum has been removed.

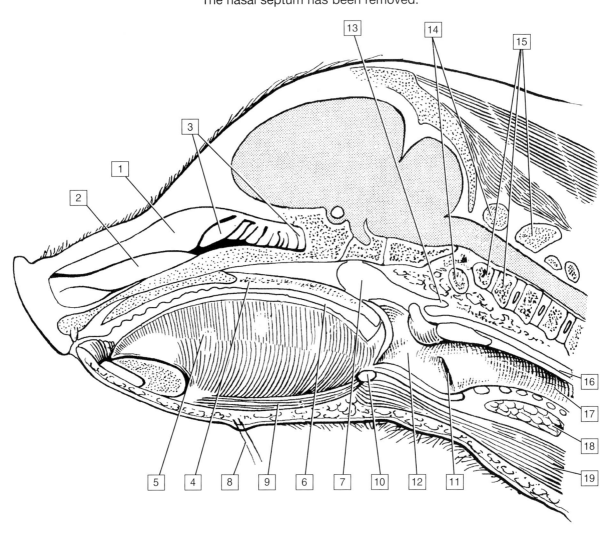

1	Dorsal nasal concha	11	Laryngeal ventricle
2	Ventral nasal concha	12	Larynx
3	Ethmoidal conchae	13	Pharyngeal diverticulum
4	Soft palate	14	Atlas
5	Tongue	15	Axis
6	Oropharynx	16	Esophagus
7	Nasopharynx	17	Trachea
8	Mental hairs	18	Thyroid gland
9	Geniohyoideus	19	Sternohyoideus
10	Basihyoid		

FIGURE 1-65

A, The development of the palate, ventral view. *B,* Transverse section through oral and nasal cavity before closure of secondary palate. *C,* Development of the tongue in the floor of the oral cavity.

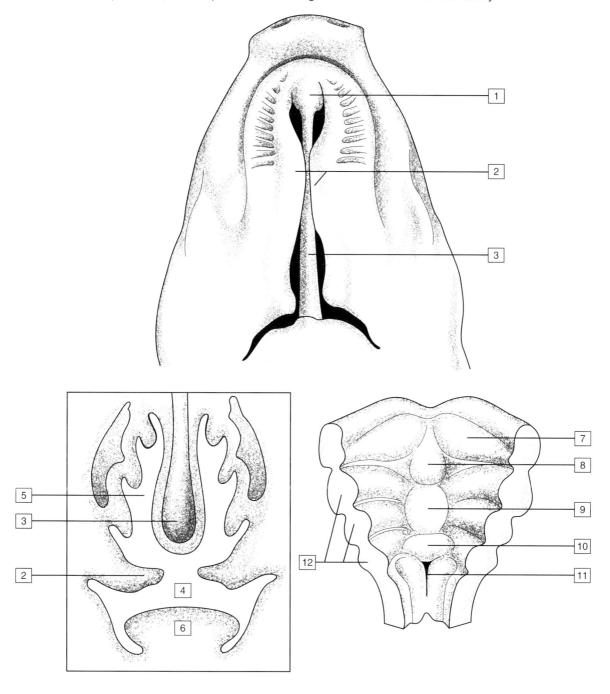

1	Primary palate	5	Nasal cavity	9	Proximal tongue swelling
2	Palatine processes (secondary palate)	6	Tongue	10	Primordium of epiglottis
3	Nasal septum	7	Distal (lateral) tongue swelling	11	Laryngeal entrance
4	Oral cavity	8	Median tongue swelling	12	Pharyngeal arches

FIGURE 1-66   Transverse Section of the Ventral Neck of Swine

A, Transverse section of the ventral neck slightly cranial to the manubrium sterni. *B,* The area within the broken line represents the topography at the slightly more caudal level of the first ribs. *C,* Pig held on its back for cranial vena cava venipuncture; see needle in position.

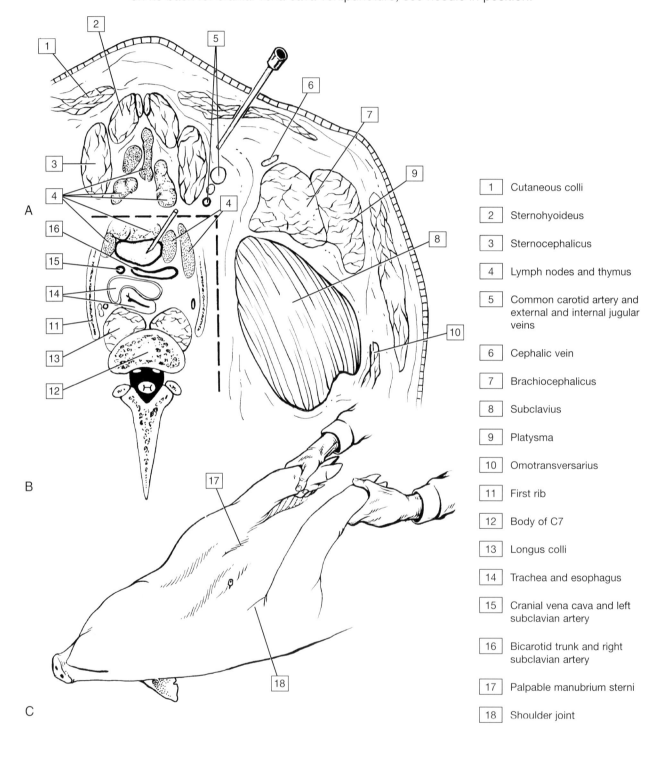

1	Cutaneous colli
2	Sternohyoideus
3	Sternocephalicus
4	Lymph nodes and thymus
5	Common carotid artery and external and internal jugular veins
6	Cephalic vein
7	Brachiocephalicus
8	Subclavius
9	Platysma
10	Omotransversarius
11	First rib
12	Body of C7
13	Longus colli
14	Trachea and esophagus
15	Cranial vena cava and left subclavian artery
16	Bicarotid trunk and right subclavian artery
17	Palpable manubrium sterni
18	Shoulder joint

FIGURE 1-67   The Lymph Centers of the Swine Head and Neck

The *arrows* indicate lymph flow.

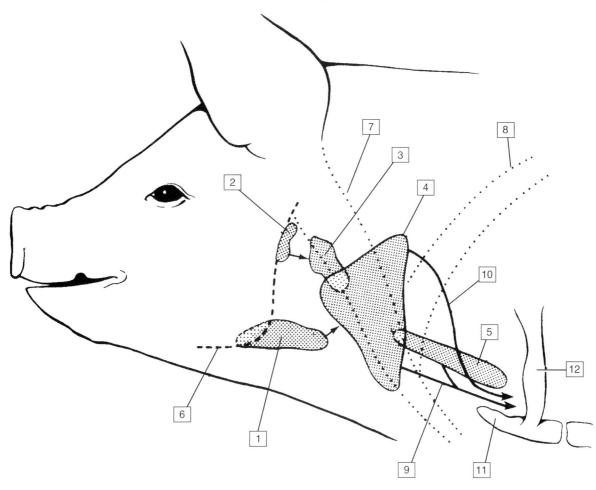

1	Mandibular lymph center	7	Brachiocephalicus
2	Parotid lymph center	8	Subclavius
3	Retropharyngeal lymph center	9	Tracheal lymph trunk
4	Superficial cervical lymph center	10	Lymph from dorsal superficial cervical nodes
5	Deep cervical lymph center	11	Manubrium sterni
6	Mandible	12	First rib

FIGURE 1-68 Avian Skull

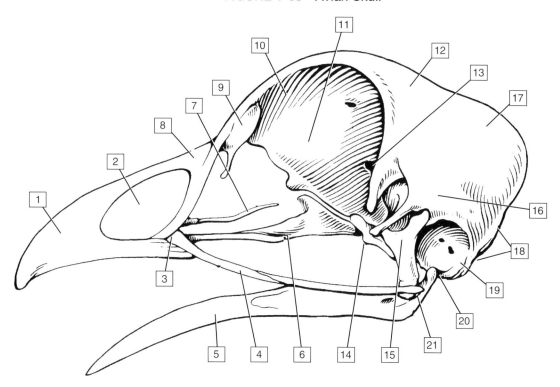

1	Premaxilla	12	Frontal bone
2	Nasal aperture	13	Optic foramen
3	Maxilla	14	Pterygoid bone
4	Jugal arch	15	Quadrate bone
5	Mandible	16	Temporal bone
6	Palatine bone	17	Parietal bone
7	Vomer	18	Occipital bone
8	Nasal bone	19	Tympanic cavity with cochlear and vestibular windows
9	Lacrimal bone	20	Sphenoid bone
10	Orbit	21	Articular bone
11	Interorbital septum		

Saunders Veterinary Anatomy Coloring Book

FIGURE 1-69   Ventral View of the Dissected Avian Neck

The inset shows a transverse section through the middle of the neck.

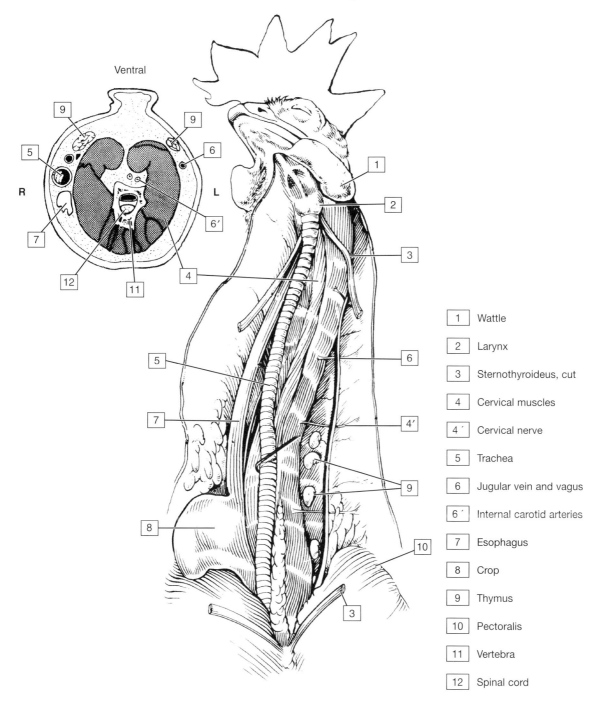

1	Wattle
2	Larynx
3	Sternothyroideus, cut
4	Cervical muscles
4´	Cervical nerve
5	Trachea
6	Jugular vein and vagus
6´	Internal carotid arteries
7	Esophagus
8	Crop
9	Thymus
10	Pectoralis
11	Vertebra
12	Spinal cord

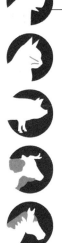

FIGURE 1-70

Dorsal view of the (A) canine, (B) feline, (C) porcine,
(D) bovine, and (E) equine tongue and epiglottis

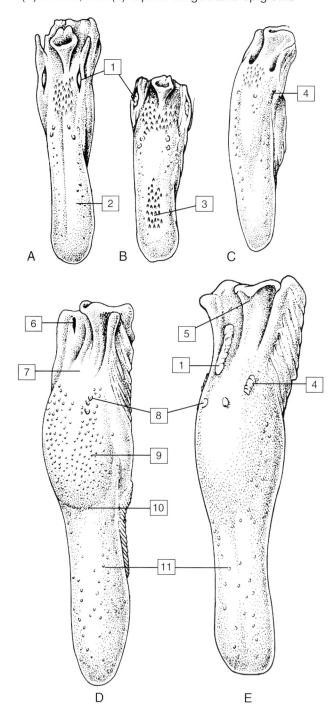

1	Palatine tonsil	4	Foliate papillae	7	Root of tongue	10	Fossa linguae
2	Median groove	5	Epiglottis	8	Vallate papillae	11	Fungiform papillae
3	Filiform papillae	6	Tonsillar sinus	9	Torus linguae		

FIGURE 1-71

Canine, porcine, bovine, and equine major salivary glands

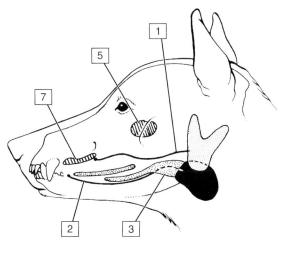

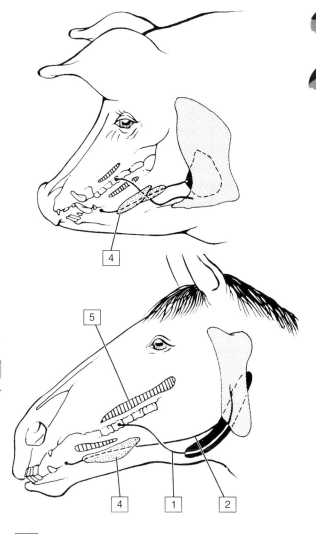

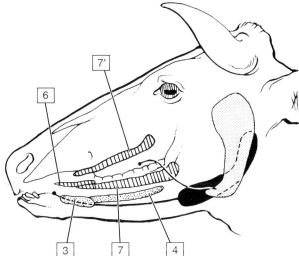

1	Parotid duct		5	Dorsal buccal glands (zygomatic gland in the dog)
2	Mandibular duct		6	Middle buccal glands
3	Compact (monostomatic) part of sublingual gland		7	Ventral buccal glands
4	Diffuse (polystomatic) part of sublingual gland		7′	Dorsal buccal gland

FIGURE 1-72

Median sections of the (A) equine, (B) bovine,
(C) porcine, and (D) canine hypophysis
The rostral extremity of the gland is to the left.

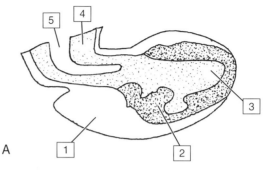

A

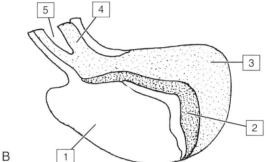

B

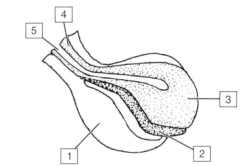

C

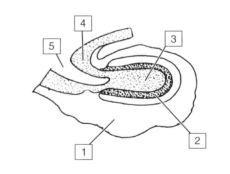

D

1	Adenohypophysis		4	Hypophysial stalk
2	Intermediate part		5	Recess of third ventricle
3	Neurohypophysis			

FIGURE 1-73 Canine and Porcine Third Eyelid

A, Left eye of dog showing third eyelid and lacrimal apparatus.
B, Isolated cartilage of the third eyelid and associated glands of a pig.

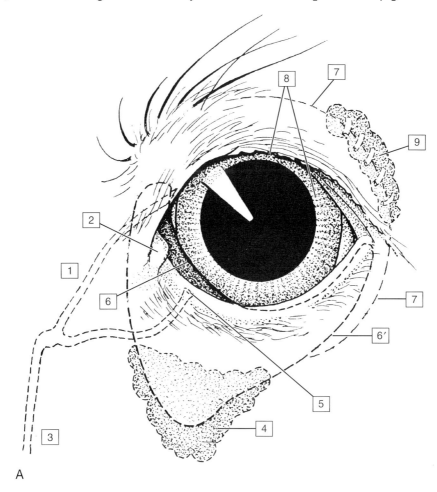

A

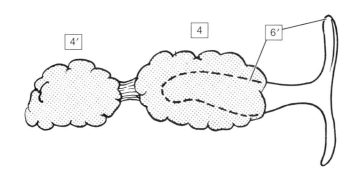

B

1	Upper canaliculus	4′	Deep gland of third eyelid	6′	Cartilage of third eyelid	9	Lacrimal gland
2	Lacrimal caruncle	5	Punctum lacrimale	7	Position of conjunctival fornix		
3	Nasolacrimal duct	6	Third eyelid	8	Pupil		
4	Gland of third eyelid						

FIGURE 2-1

Transection of the canine vertebral
column to show the formation of a spinal nerve

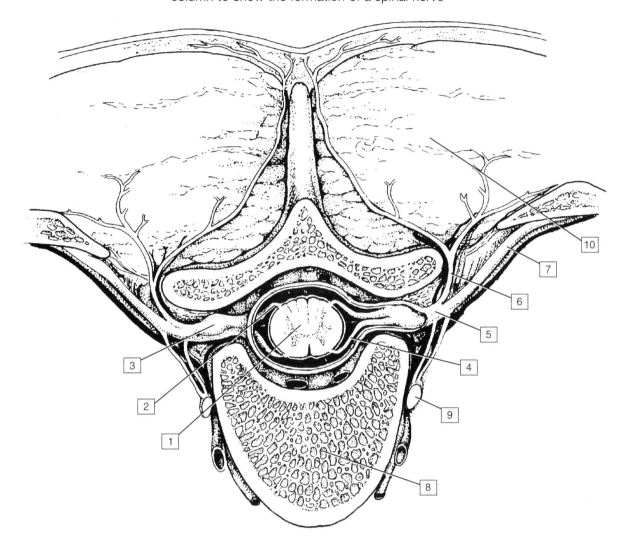

1	Spinal cord	6	Dorsal branch of spinal nerve
2	Dorsal root	7	Ventral branch of spinal nerve
3	Spinal ganglion	8	Body of vertebra
4	Ventral root	9	Sympathetic trunk
5	Spinal nerve	10	Epaxial muscles

FIGURE 2-2   Cervical and Thoracic Vertebrae of the Dog

A, Axis, lateral view. *B,* Fifth vertebra, lateral
view. *C,* Thoracic vertebra, left lateral view.

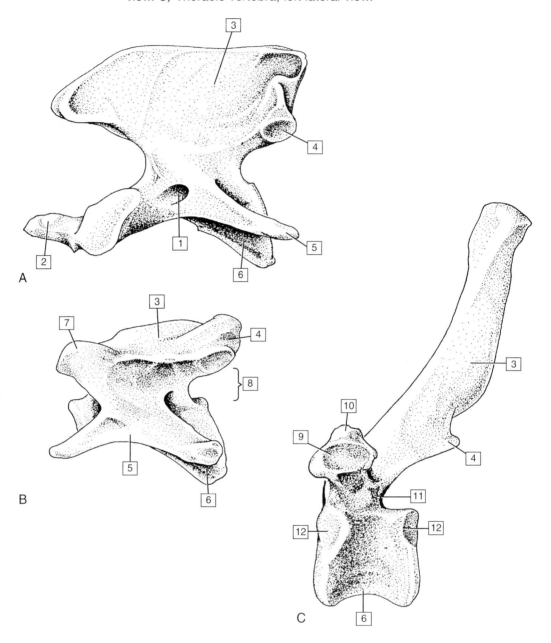

1	Transverse foramen	7	Cranial articular process
2	Dens	8	Position of vertebral foramen
3	Spinous process	9	Transverse process with costal fovea
4	Caudal articular process	10	Mammillary process
5	Transverse process	11	Caudal vertebral notch
6	Body	12	Costal foveae

FIGURE 2-3 Dorsal Roots of Spinal Nerves and Spinal Cord Segments

Dorsal view, vertebral arches removed. Dura removed on left side of both figures.

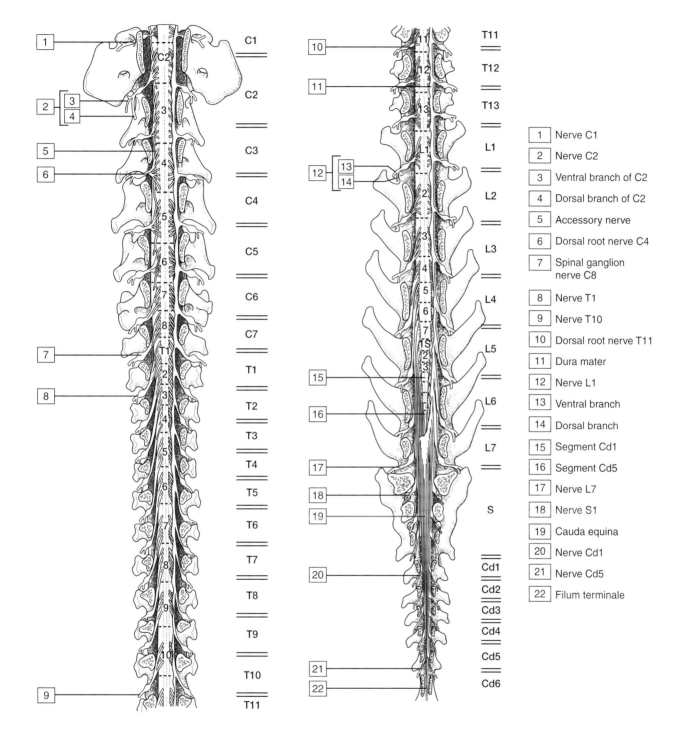

1	Nerve C1
2	Nerve C2
3	Ventral branch of C2
4	Dorsal branch of C2
5	Accessory nerve
6	Dorsal root nerve C4
7	Spinal ganglion nerve C8
8	Nerve T1
9	Nerve T10
10	Dorsal root nerve T11
11	Dura mater
12	Nerve L1
13	Ventral branch
14	Dorsal branch
15	Segment Cd1
16	Segment Cd5
17	Nerve L7
18	Nerve S1
19	Cauda equina
20	Nerve Cd1
21	Nerve Cd5
22	Filum terminale

FIGURE 2-4 Schematic View of Terminal Spinal Cord with Dura Reflected

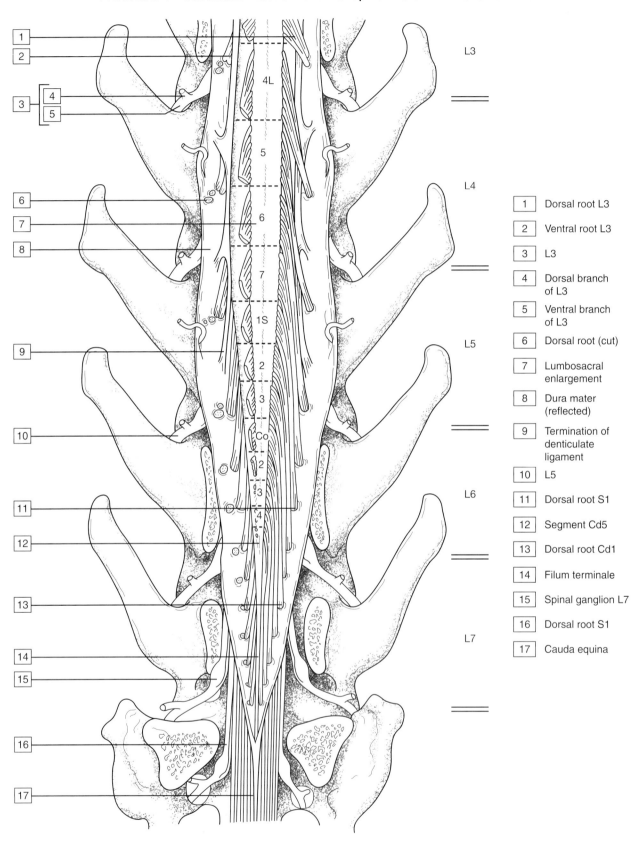

1	Dorsal root L3
2	Ventral root L3
3	L3
4	Dorsal branch of L3
5	Ventral branch of L3
6	Dorsal root (cut)
7	Lumbosacral enlargement
8	Dura mater (reflected)
9	Termination of denticulate ligament
10	L5
11	Dorsal root S1
12	Segment Cd5
13	Dorsal root Cd1
14	Filum terminale
15	Spinal ganglion L7
16	Dorsal root S1
17	Cauda equina

FIGURE 2-5   Ventral Muscles of the Canine Neck and Thorax

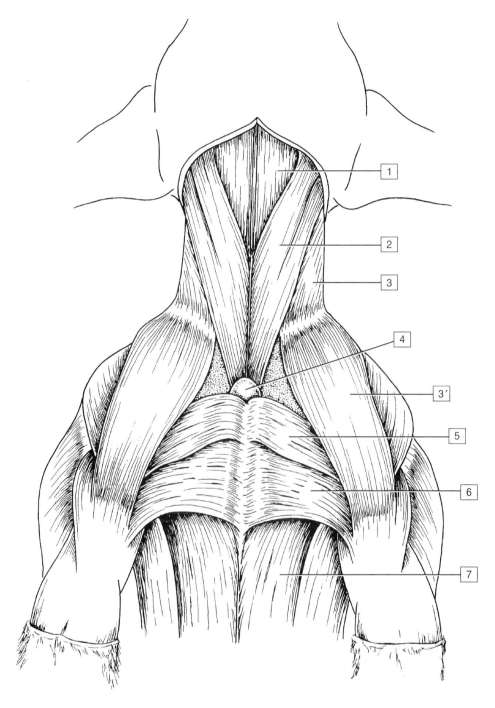

1	Combined sternohyoideus and sternothyroideus	4	Manubrium of sternum
2	Sternocephalicus	5	Pectoralis descendens
3	Brachiocephalicus: cleidocervicalis	6	Pectoralis transversus
3'	Brachiocephalicus: cleidobrachialis	7	Pectoralis profundus

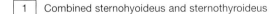

Saunders Veterinary Anatomy Coloring Book

FIGURE 2-6   Transverse Section of the Canine
Back at the Level of the First Lumbar Vertebra

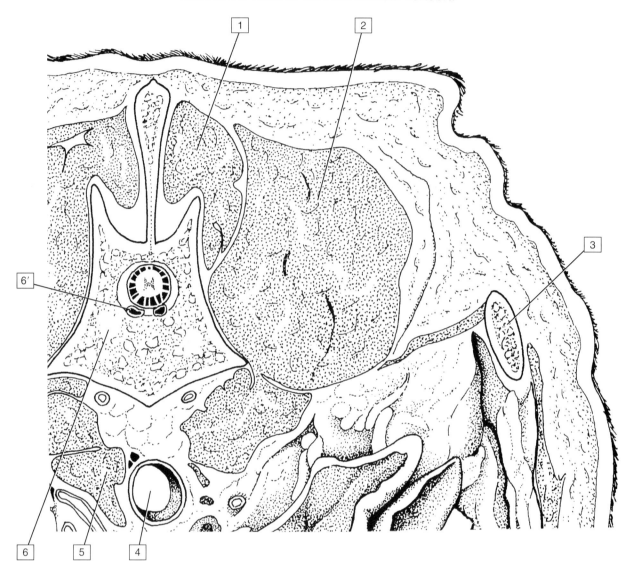

1	Multifidus and spinalis	5	Right crus of diaphragm
2	Longissimus and iliocostalis	6	First lumbar vertebra
3	Last rib	6′	Internal vertebral venous plexus
4	Aorta		

FIGURE 2-7   Muscles Associated with the Canine
Atlantooccipital and Atlantoaxial Joints, Lateral View

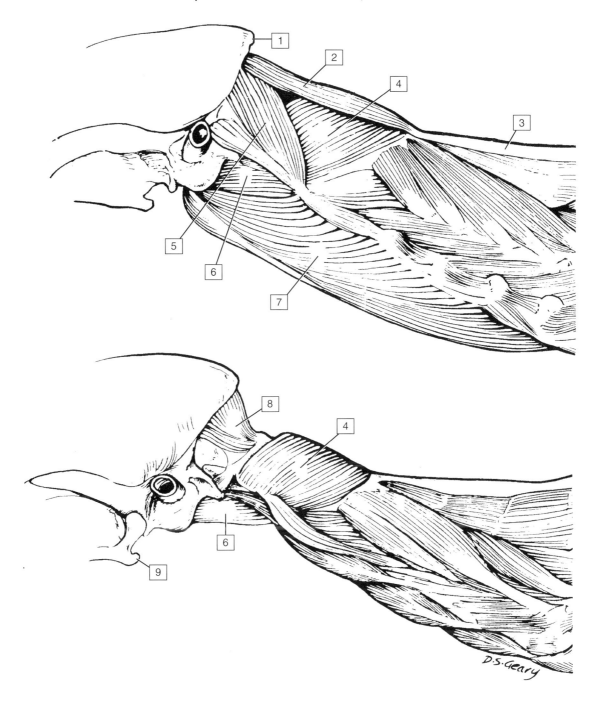

1	External occipital protuberance	6	Rectus capitis ventralis
2	Rectus capitis dorsalis major	7	Longus capitis
3	Nuchal ligament	8	Rectus capitis dorsalis minor
4	Obliquus capitis caudalis	9	Angular process of mandible
5	Obliquus capitis cranialis		

FIGURE 2-8 Peripheral Distribution of Canine
Sympathetic and Parasympathetic Divisions

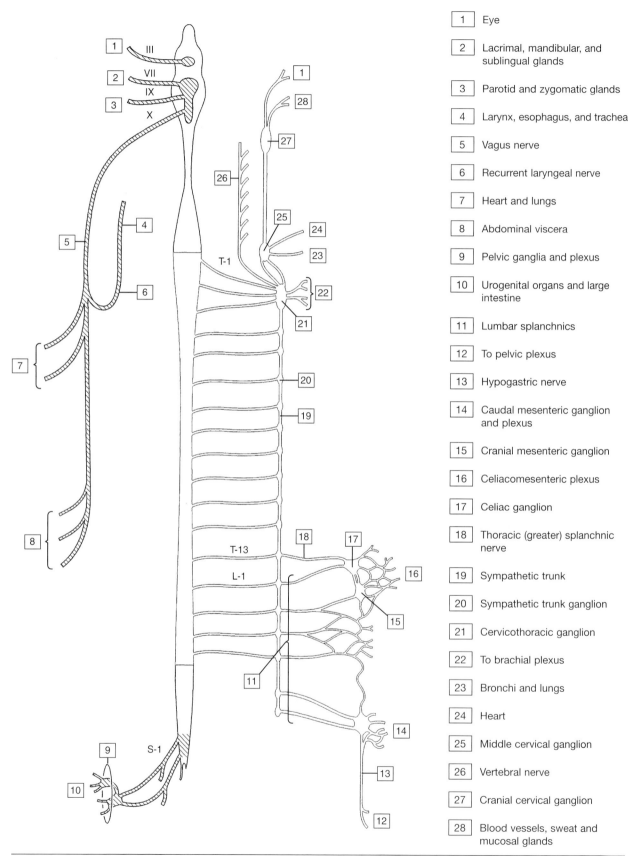

1	Eye
2	Lacrimal, mandibular, and sublingual glands
3	Parotid and zygomatic glands
4	Larynx, esophagus, and trachea
5	Vagus nerve
6	Recurrent laryngeal nerve
7	Heart and lungs
8	Abdominal viscera
9	Pelvic ganglia and plexus
10	Urogenital organs and large intestine
11	Lumbar splanchnics
12	To pelvic plexus
13	Hypogastric nerve
14	Caudal mesenteric ganglion and plexus
15	Cranial mesenteric ganglion
16	Celiacomesenteric plexus
17	Celiac ganglion
18	Thoracic (greater) splanchnic nerve
19	Sympathetic trunk
20	Sympathetic trunk ganglion
21	Cervicothoracic ganglion
22	To brachial plexus
23	Bronchi and lungs
24	Heart
25	Middle cervical ganglion
26	Vertebral nerve
27	Cranial cervical ganglion
28	Blood vessels, sweat and mucosal glands

FIGURE 2-9   Canine Epaxial Muscles

Each of the named muscles shown can be present, spanning other
vertebrae, thus overlapping and obscuring their individual nature.

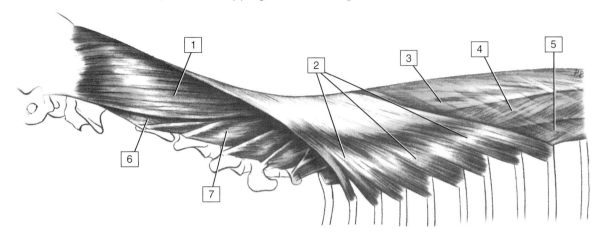

1	Splenius	5	Iliocostalis
2	Serratus dorsalis cranialis	6	Longissimus capitis
3	Spinalis at semispinalis	7	Longissimus cervicis
4	Longissimus		

FIGURE 2-10   Equine Sternum and Costal Cartilages, Lateral View

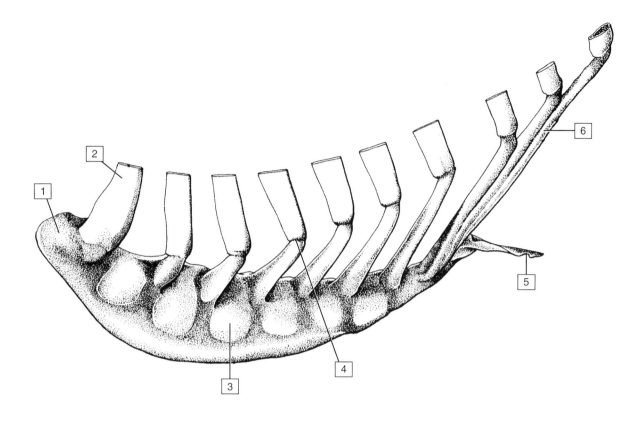

1	Manubrium	4	Costochondral junction
2	First rib	5	Xiphoid cartilage
3	Sternebra	6	Costal arch

Saunders Veterinary Anatomy Coloring Book

FIGURE 2-11   Superficial Dissection of the Equine Head

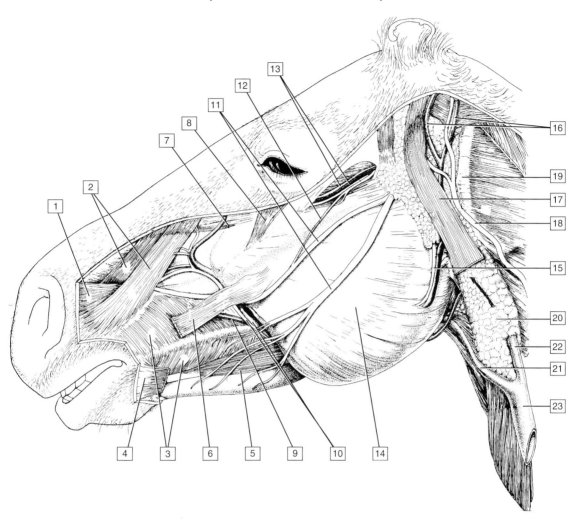

1 Caninus	9 Parotid duct	16 Auricular veins
2 Levator nasolabialis	10 Facial artery and vein	17 Parotid auricularis
3 Buccinator	11 Buccal branches of facial nerve	18 Great auricular nerve (C2)
4 Stump of cutaneous muscle joining orbicularis oris	12 Rostral communicating branch of auriculotemporal nerve	19 Wing of atlas
5 Depressor labii inferioris	13 Transverse facial artery and vein and transverse facial branch of auriculotemporal nerve	20 Parotid gland
6 Zygomaticus		21 Linguofacial vein
7 Levator labii superioris	14 Masseter	22 Maxillary vein
8 Malaris	15 Masseteric artery and vein	23 External jugular vein

FIGURE 2-12 Segmentation of the Bovine Paraxial Mesoderm

10-mm bovine embryo (*top*) together with two stages in the development
of the vertebrae and related vessels and nerves. The *arrows* show
the formation of each vertebra from two pairs of adjacent somites.

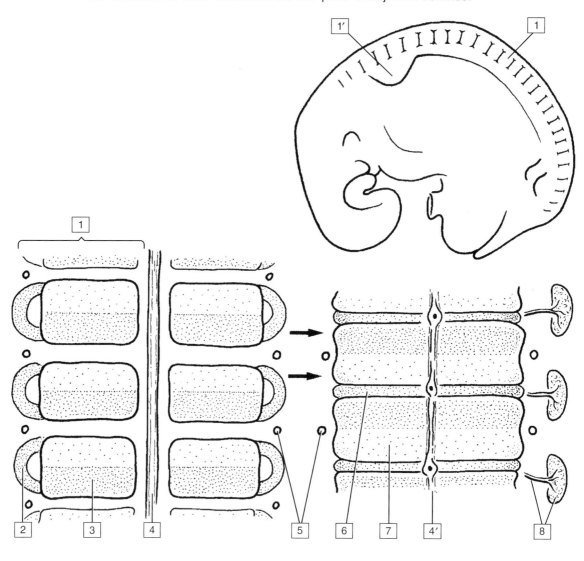

1	Somite	5	Intersegmental artery
1'	Forelimb bud	6	Intervertebral disc
2	Myotome	7	Body of vertebra
3	Sclerotome	8	Myotome with segmental nerve
4	Notochord		
4'	Notochord giving rise to the nucleus pulposus in the center of the intervertebral disc (6)		

FIGURE 2-13 Caudal Part of the Bovine Vertebral Canal and Its Contents

Epidural injection sites are indicated by the needles.

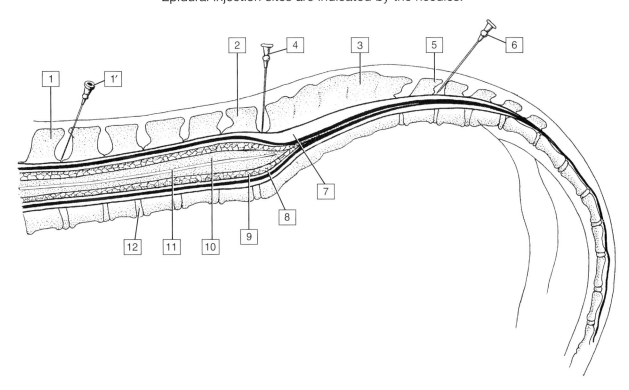

1	First lumbar vertebra	7	Epidural space
1′	Needle in position for flank anesthesia	8	Dura mater
2	Last lumbar vertebra (L6)	9	Subarachnoid space
3	Sacrum	10	Spinal cord
4	Needle in lumbosacral space	11	Central canal
5	First caudal vertebra	12	Intervertebral disc
6	Needle between first and second caudal vertebrae (tail block)		

FIGURE 2-14   The Connections of the Major Veins with
the Bovine Vertebral Plexus-Azygous System

Note, specifically, the connections between the internal vertebral plexus and the
intercostal veins and between the plexus and the branches of the vertebral vein.

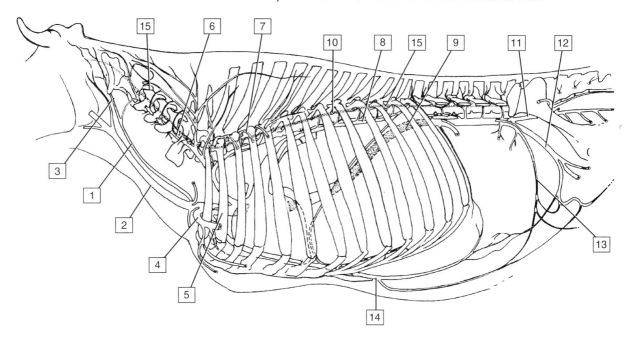

1	Internal jugular v.		9	Caudal vena cava
2	External jugular v.		10	Intercostal v.
3	Occipital v.		11	Internal iliac v.
4	Axillary v.		12	External iliac v.
5	Second rib		13	Deep circumflex iliac v.
6	Vertebral v.		14	Cranial epigastric v.
7	Supreme intercostal v.		15	Internal vertebral plexus, stippled in the vertebral canal
8	Left azygous v.			

FIGURE 2-15   Avian Uropygial (Preen) Gland, Dorsal View

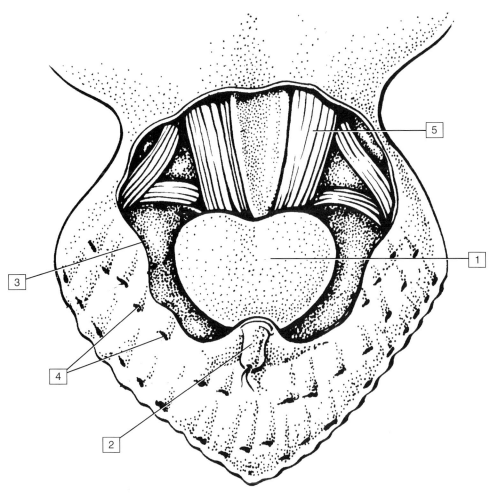

1	Uropygial gland	4	Feather follicles
2	Papilla of uropygial gland through which the secretion is extruded	5	Caudal vertebrae and associated muscles
3	Cut edge of skin		

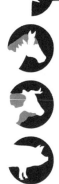

FIGURE 2-16 The Canine *(A)*, Equine *(B)*, Bovine *(C)*, and Porcine *(D)* Thyroid Gland

The inset to *D* illustrates the subtracheal connection in transverse section in the pig.

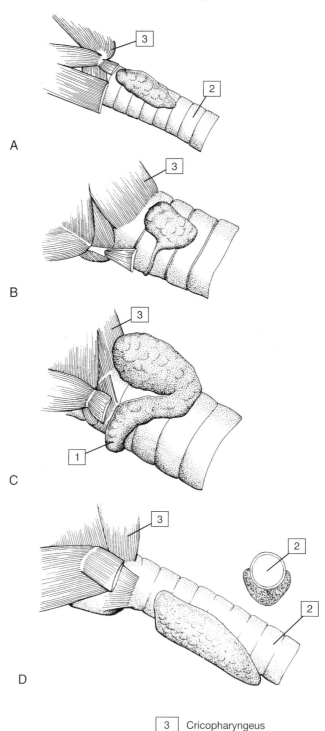

A

B

C

D

1	Isthmus	
2	Trachea	
3	Cricopharyngeus	

THE THORAX

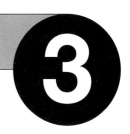

FIGURE 3-1 Schematic View of the Partitioning of the Atrium and Ventricle

A, The primary atrial septum has formed, and development of the interventricular septum has begun. *B,* The primary atrial septum has fused with the endocardial cushions, and a secondary foramen (5) has been formed. *C,* The secondary atrial septum has formed, and a passage (foramen ovale) between primary and secondary septa connects the right and left atria. Note the fusion of the interventricular septum with the endocardial cushions.

Note: This is a generic representation of a heart and does not pertain to any particular species.

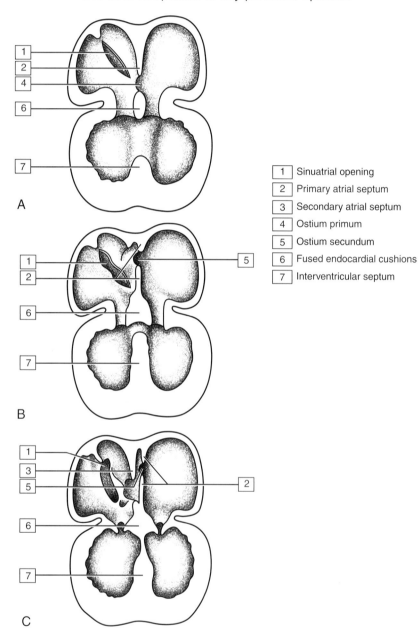

1	Sinuatrial opening
2	Primary atrial septum
3	Secondary atrial septum
4	Ostium primum
5	Ostium secundum
6	Fused endocardial cushions
7	Interventricular septum

FIGURE 3-2   Schema of Canine Circulation

Vessels carrying oxygenated blood are shown in white,
and those carrying deoxygenated blood are shown in black.

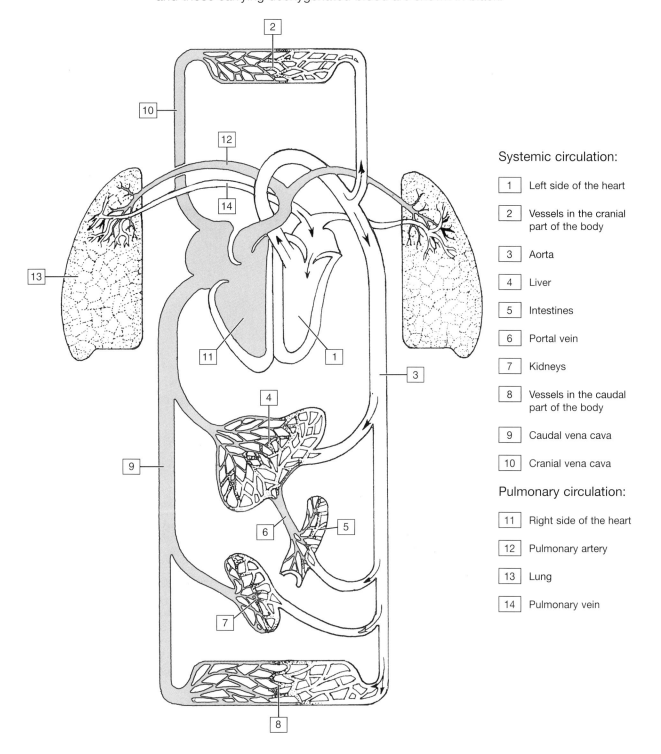

Systemic circulation:

1	Left side of the heart
2	Vessels in the cranial part of the body
3	Aorta
4	Liver
5	Intestines
6	Portal vein
7	Kidneys
8	Vessels in the caudal part of the body
9	Caudal vena cava
10	Cranial vena cava

Pulmonary circulation:

11	Right side of the heart
12	Pulmonary artery
13	Lung
14	Pulmonary vein

FIGURE 3-3 Canine Trunk Muscles, Deeper Layers

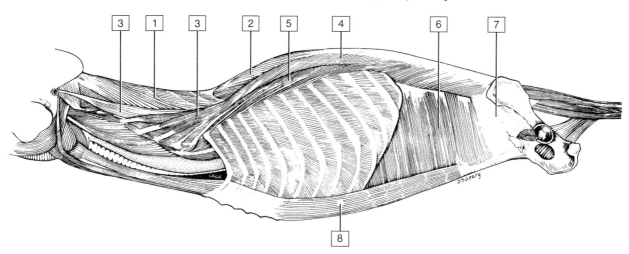

1	Semispinalis capitis	
2	Spinalis et semispinalis	
3	Longissimus capitis and cervicis	
4	Longissimus thoracis	

5	Iliocostalis	
6	Transversus abdominis	
7	Transverse fascia	
8	Rectus abdominis	

Saunders Veterinary Anatomy Coloring Book

FIGURE 3-4   Canine Trunk Muscles, Deepest Layers

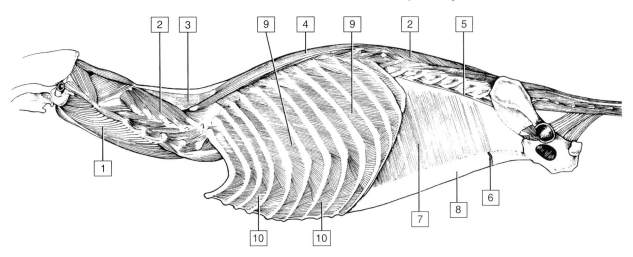

1 Longus capitis	6 Rectus abdominis
2 Multifidus	7 Transversus abdominis
3 Spinalis cervicis	8 Aponeurosis of transversus abdominis
4 Spinalis et semispinalis	9 External intercostal muscles
5 Quadratus lumborum	10 Internal intercostal muscles

FIGURE 3-5   Muscular Suspension of the
Canine Thorax between the Forelimbs

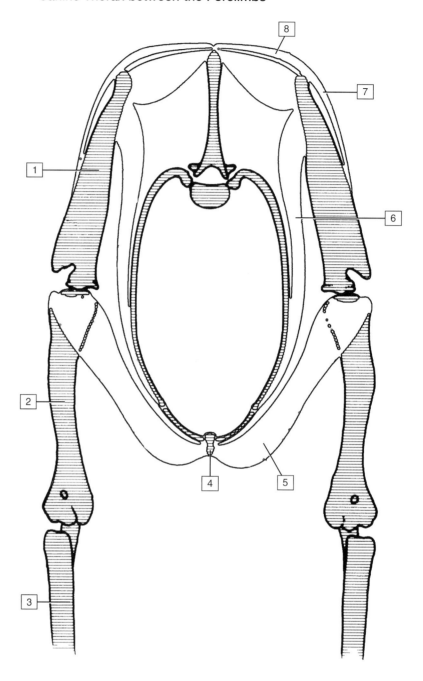

1	Scapula	5	Pectoralis profundus (ascendens)
2	Humerus	6	Serratus ventralis
3	Radius and ulna	7	Trapezius
4	Sternum	8	Rhomboideus

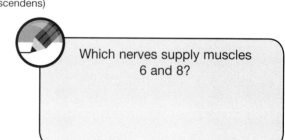

Which nerves supply muscles
6 and 8?

Saunders Veterinary Anatomy Coloring Book

FIGURE 3-6   The Distribution of the Canine Pleura and Pericardium

The heavy lines indicate the pleura.

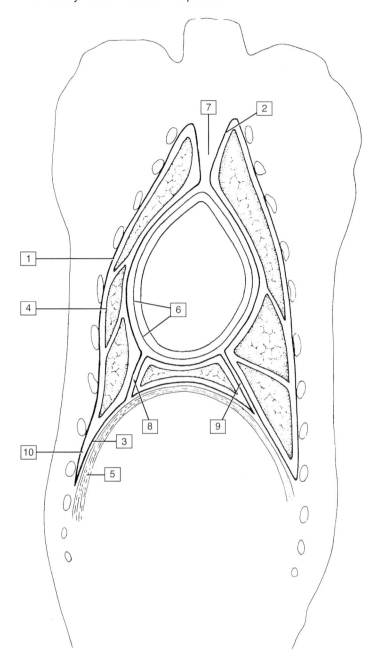

1	Costal pleura	7	Cranial mediastinum
2	Mediastinal pleura	8	Caudal mediastinum
3	Diaphragmatic pleura	9	Plica venae cavae
4	Visceral pleura	10	Costodiaphragmatic recess
5	Diaphragm		
6	Parietal pericardium; its outer fibrous layer tightly adheres to its inner serous layer		

FIGURE 3-7   Section of the Canine Heart Exposing the Four Chambers

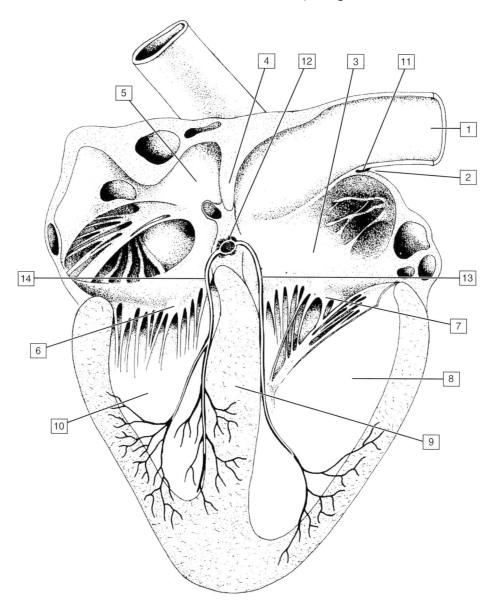

1	Cranial vena cava	
2	Terminal sulcus	
3	Right atrium	
4	Interatrial septum	
5	Left atrium	
6	Left atrioventricular valve	
7	Right atrioventricular valve	
8	Right ventricle	
9	Interventricular septum	
10	Left ventricle	
11	Sinoatrial node	
12	Atrioventricular node	
13	Right and left limbs of atrioventricular bundle	
14	Right and left limbs of atrioventricular bundle	

Draw the impulse conduction pathway on this figure.

Saunders Veterinary Anatomy Coloring Book

FIGURE 3-8 Canine Pericardium

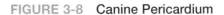
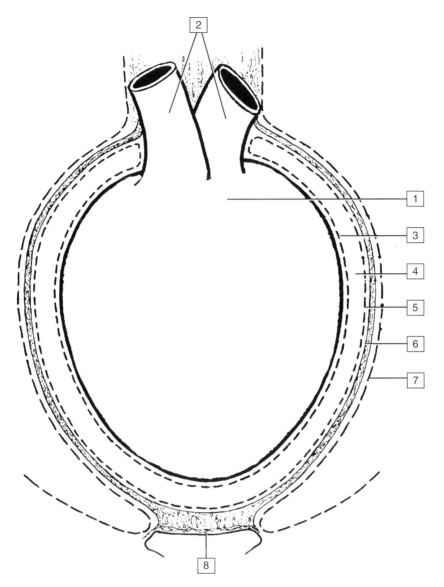

1	Heart		5	Parietal pericardium
2	Great vessels		6	Connective tissue layer of the parietal pericardium
3	Visceral pericardium (epicardium)		7	Mediastinal pleura
4	Pericardial cavity (exaggerated in size)		8	Sternopericardial ligament

FIGURE 3-9   Canine Cardiac Nerves and Related Ganglia Left Lateral View

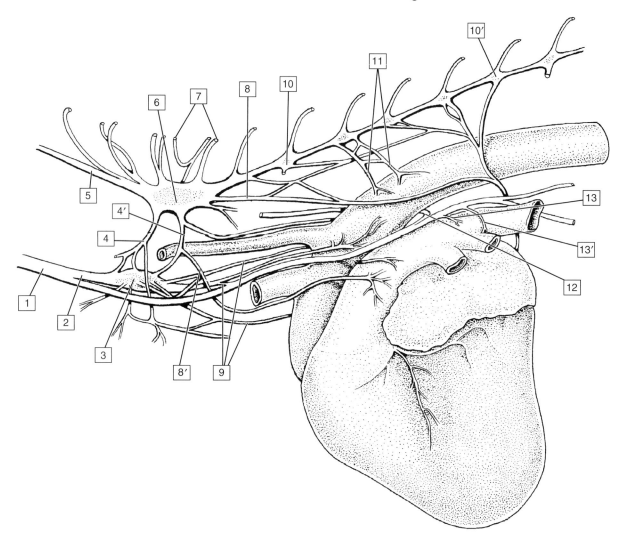

1	Vagosympathetic trunk	8'	Caudoventral cervicothoracic cardiac n.
2	Sympathetic trunk	9	Vertebral cardiac n.
3	Middle cervical ganglion	10	Third thoracic ganglion
4	Cranial limb of ansa subclavia	10'	Seventh thoracic ganglion
4'	Caudal limb of ansa subclavia	11	Thoracic cardiac n.
5	Vertebral n.	12	Left recurrent laryngeal n.
6	Cervicothoracic ganglion	13	Cranial vagal cardiac n.
7	Communicating branches	13'	Caudal vagal cardiac n.
8	Caudodorsal cervicothoracic cardiac n.		

Saunders Veterinary Anatomy Coloring Book

FIGURE 3-10   The Components of the Canine Arterial Wall

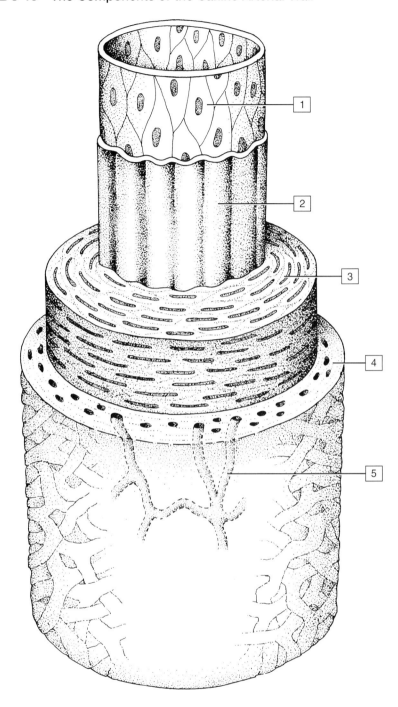

1	Endothelium
2	Inner elastic membrane
3	Tunica media

| 4 | Tunica adventitia |
| 5 | Vasa vasorum |

FIGURE 3-11   Branching of the Canine Aortic Arch

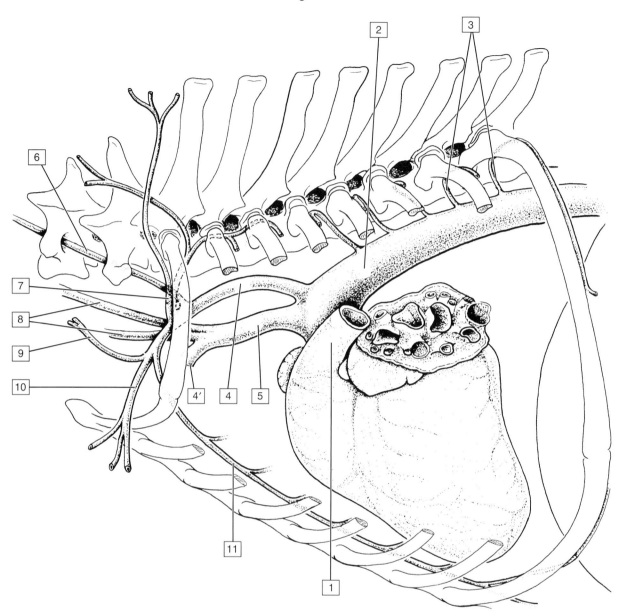

1	Pulmonary trunk	6	Vertebral a.
2	Aorta	7	Costocervical trunk
3	Intercostal aa.	8	Left and right common carotid aa.
4'	Left subclavian a.	9	Superficial cervical a.
4	Right subclavian a.	10	Axillary a.
5	Brachiocephalic trunk	11	Internal thoracic a.

FIGURE 3-12   The Canine Fetal *(A)* and Postnatal *(B)* Circulatory Systems

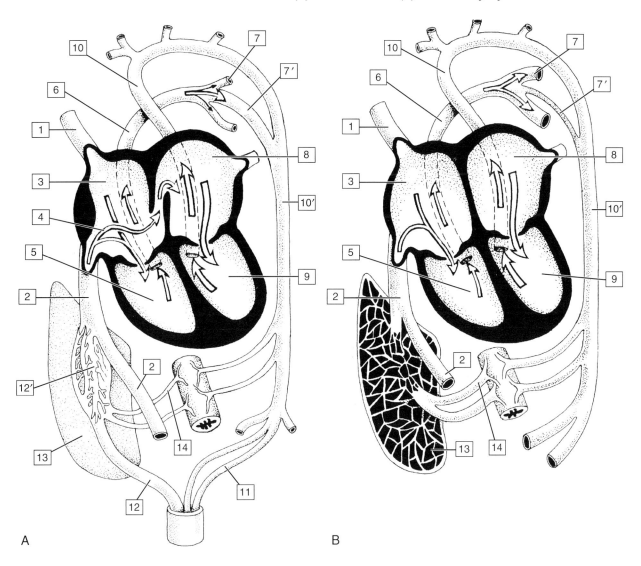

A

B

1	Cranial vena cava		9	Left ventricle
2	Caudal vena cava		10	Aortic arch
3	Right atrium		10'	Descending aorta
4	Arrow entering oval foramen		11	Umbilical artery
5	Right ventricle		12	Umbilical vein
6	Pulmonary trunk		12'	Ductus venosus
7	Pulmonary artery		13	Liver
7'	Ductus arteriosus (in *B*, vestige)		14	Portal vein
8	Left atrium			

FIGURE 3-13   Lymph Drainage of the Canine Lumbosacral Area Ventral View

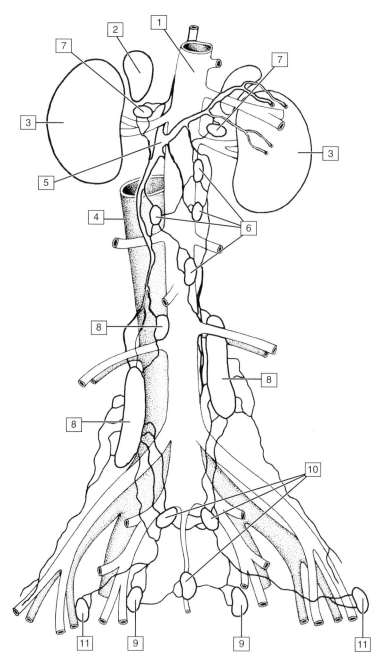

1	Aorta	7	Renal nodes
2	Adrenals	8	Medial iliac nodes
3	Kidneys	9	Hypogastric nodes
4	Caudal vena cava	10	Sacral nodes
5	Cisterna chyli	11	Deep inguinal (iliofemoral) nodes
6	Lumbar aortic nodes		

FIGURE 3-14 Vessels on the Floor of the Canine Thorax

The transversus thoracis has been removed on the right.

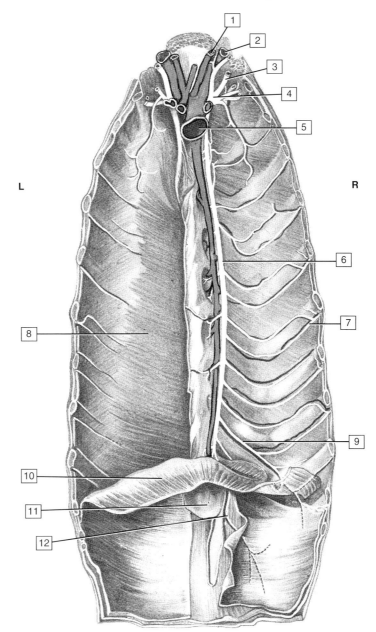

L

R

1	Internal jugular vein	7	Intercostal artery
2	External jugular vein	8	Transversus thoracis
3	Vertebral artery	9	Musculophrenic artery
4	Right subclavian artery	10	Diaphragm
5	Cranial vena cava	11	Xiphoid cartilage
6	Internal thoracic artery	12	Cranial epigastric artery

FIGURE 3-15 Muscles of the Canine Neck and Thorax, Lateral View

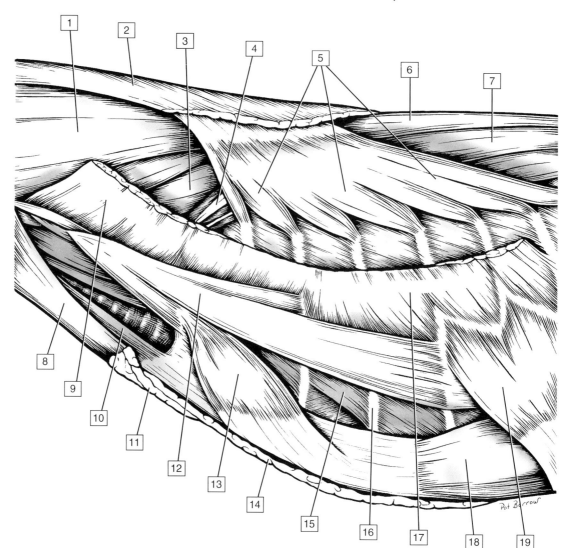

1	Splenius
2	Rhomboideus
3	Longissimus cervicis
4	Longissimus thoracis
5	Serratus dorsalis cranialis
6	Spinalis and semispinalis thoracis
7	Longissimus thoracis
8	Sternocephalicus
9	Serratus ventralis (cervicis)
10	Sternothyroideus
11	Superficial pectoral
12	Scalenus
13	Rectus thoracis
14	Deep pectoral
15	External intercostal muscle
16	Fourth rib
17	Serratus ventralis (thoracis)
18	Rectus abdominis
19	External abdominal oblique

FIGURE 3-16   Left and Right Surface Projections of the Feline Heart and Lung

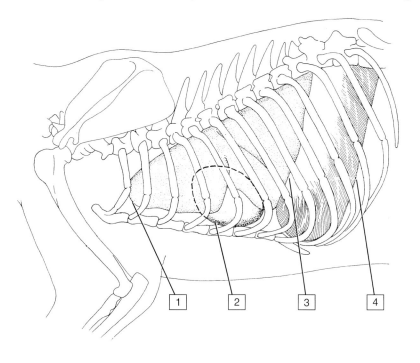

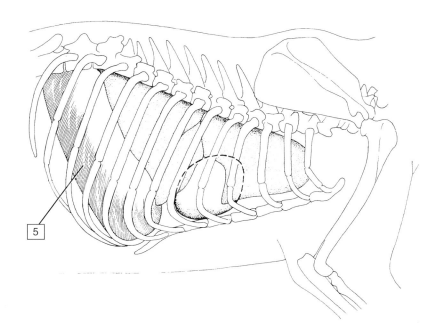

1	Apex of left lung	4	Line of pleural reflection
2	Heart	5	Diaphragm
3	Basal border of lung		

Draw the pulmonary and right artrio-ventricular valves on the figures.

FIGURE 3-17 Projections of the Equine Heart
and Lung on the Left and Right Thoracic Walls

The heavy line indicates the caudal border of the triceps.

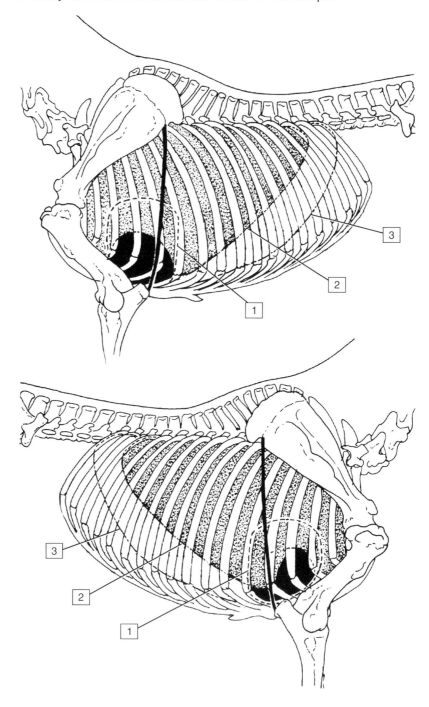

1	Outline of heart	3	Line of pleural reflection
2	Basal border of lung		

FIGURE 3-18   Left Lateral View of the Bovine Thoracic Cavity

The left lung and part of the mediastinal pleura have been removed.

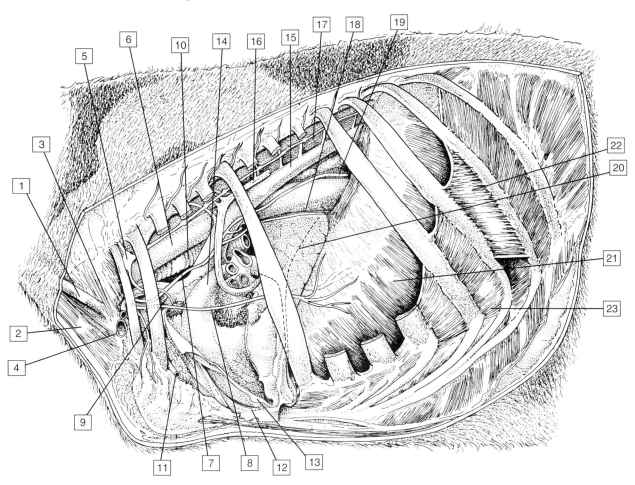

1	External jugular vein	13	Pericardium, reflected
2	Sternocephalicus	14	Pulmonary trunk
3	Axillary artery	15	Aorta
4	Axillary vein	16	Left azygous vein
5	Cervicothoracic ganglion	17	Greater splanchnic nerve
6	Esophagus	18	Ventral vagal trunk
7	Vagus	19	Dorsal vagal trunk
8	Phrenic nerve	20	Cranial extent of diaphragm
9	One of the cardiac nerves	21	Diaphragm
10	Trachea	22	Internal intercostal muscle
11	Internal thoracic artery	23	External intercostal muscle
12	Mediastinal pleura		

FIGURE 3-19 Base of the Bovine Heart
(Atria has been Removed), Dorsal View

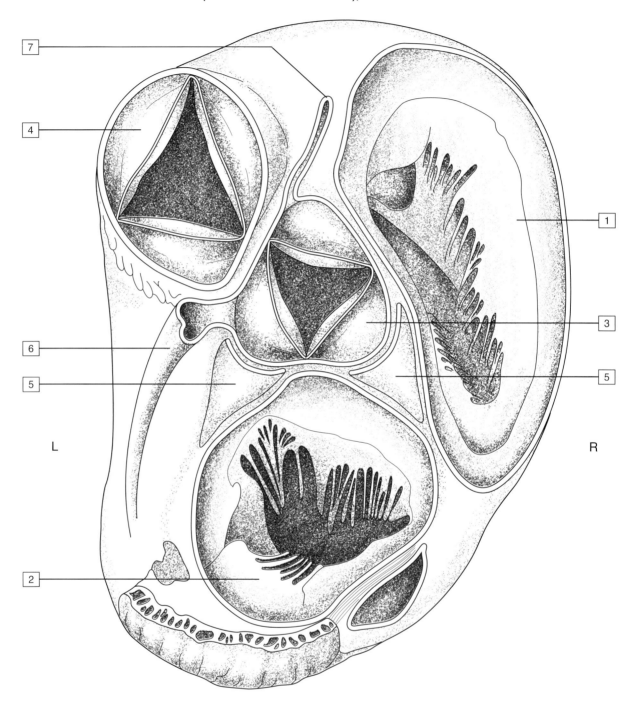

L

R

1	Right atrioventricular valve	5	Ossa cordis
2	Left atrioventricular valve	6	Left coronary artery
3	Aortic valve	7	Right coronary artery
4	Pulmonary valve		

Saunders Veterinary Anatomy Coloring Book

FIGURE 3-20   Lobation and Bronchial Tree
of the Bovine Lungs, Schematic Dorsal View

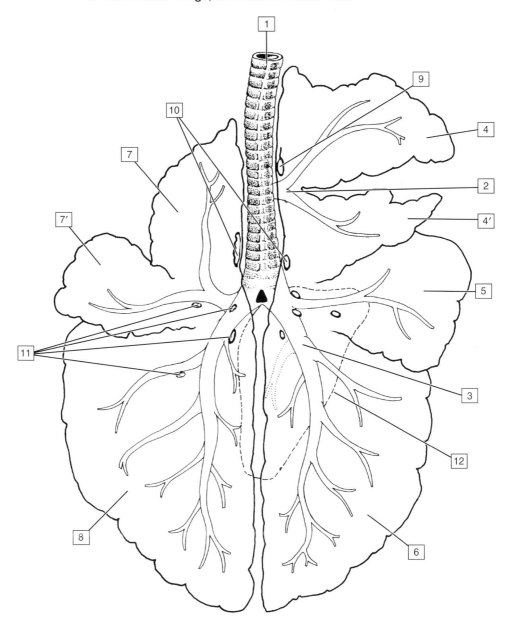

1	Trachea	7	Divided left cranial bone
2	Tracheal bronchus	7'	Divided left cranial lobe
3	Right principal bronchus	8	Left caudal lobe
4	Divided right cranial lobe	9	Cranial tracheobronchial lymph node
4'	Divided right cranial lobe	10	Tracheobronchial lymph nodes
5	Middle lobe	11	Pulmonary lymph nodes
6	Right caudal lobe	12	Outline of accessory lobe of right lung

FIGURE 3-21   Porcine Embryo after Fusion of the Endocardial Tube

A, Ventral view of the cranial part of a 15-day-old pig embryo
after fusion of the endocardial tube. *B*, Transverse section of
a seven- to eight-somite embryo taken at the level of 5.

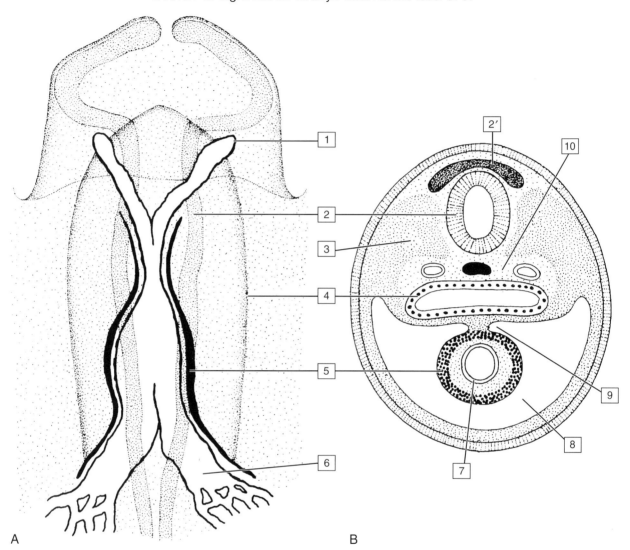

A

B

1	First aortic arch	6	Vitelline vein
2	Neural tube	7	Endocardial tube
2'	Neural crest	8	Pericardial cavity
3	Somite	9	Dorsal mesocardium
4	Foregut	10	Notochord and dorsal aortae
5	Epimyocardial wall of the fused endocardial tubes		

Saunders Veterinary Anatomy Coloring Book

FIGURE 3-22   Porcine Heart in situ

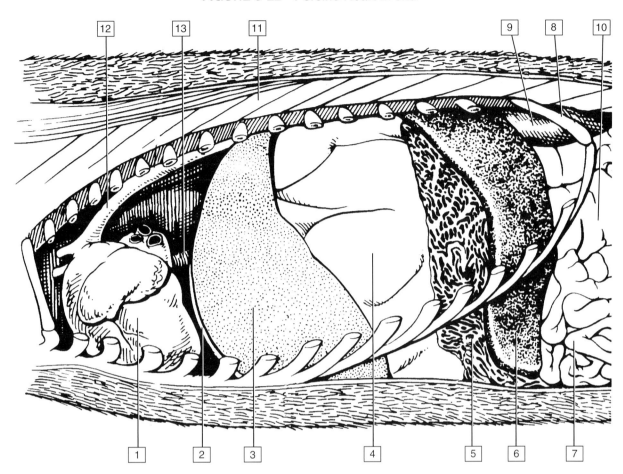

1	Heart	8	Last rib
2	Diaphragm	9	Left kidney
3	Left lobe of liver	10	Ascending colon
4	Stomach, greatly dilated	11	Back muscles
5	Greater omentum, gastrosplenic ligament	12	Aorta
6	Spleen	13	Caudal vena cava
7	Jejunum		

FIGURE 3-23   Porcine Lymph Centers of the Thorax, Left Lateral View

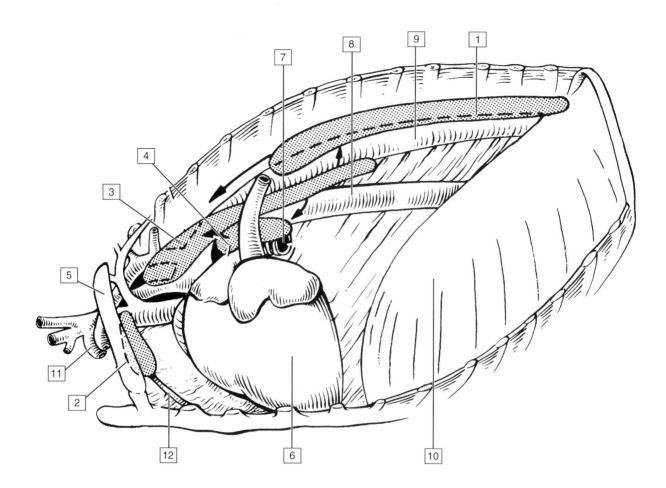

1	Dorsal thoracic lymph center	
2	Ventral thoracic lymph center	
3	Mediastinal lymph center	
4	Tracheobronchial lymph center	
5	First rib	
6	Heart	

7	Left bronchus	
8	Esophagus	
9	Aorta	
10	Diaphragm	
11	Axillary vein and artery	
12	Internal thoracic artery	

Saunders Veterinary Anatomy Coloring Book

FIGURE 3-24   Avian Flight Muscles, Dissected and Shown in Ventral View

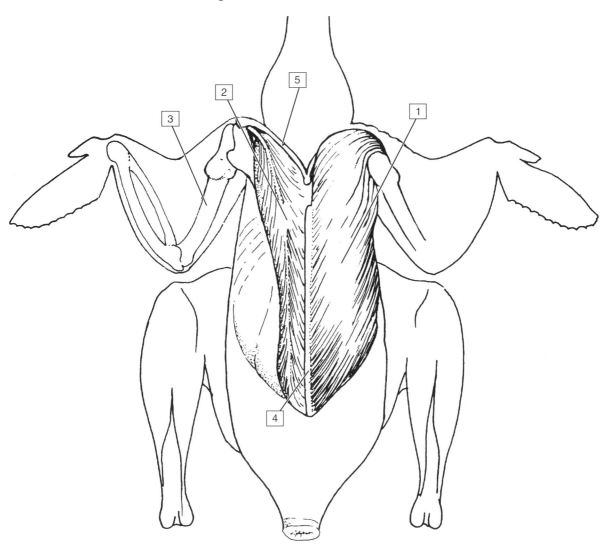

1	Pectoralis	4	Sternum
2	Supracoracoideus	5	Clavicle
3	Humerus		

FIGURE 3-25   **Right Avian Lung (Medioventral View) and Related Air Sacs**

The intrapulmonic structures have been simplified.

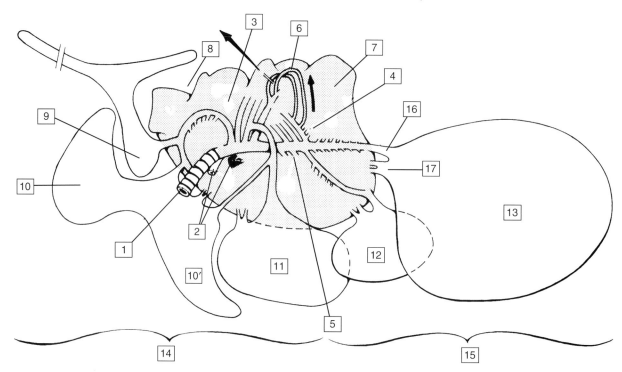

1	Primary bronchus	**10'**	Extrathoracic and intrathoracic parts of clavicular air sac
2	Pulmonary vessels at hilus	**11**	Cranial thoracic air sac
3	Medioventral bronchi	**12**	Caudal thoracic air sac
4	Mediodorsal bronchi	**13**	Abdominal air sac
5	Lateroventral bronchi	**14**	Cranial air sacs, functionally related to paleopulmonic parabronchi
6	Loops of parabronchi		
7	Lung	**15**	Caudal air sacs, functionally related to neopulmonic parabronchi
8	Indentations caused by ribs		
9	Cervical air sac	**16**	Direct (saccobronchial) connection
10	Extrathoracic and intrathoracic parts of clavicular air sac	**17**	Indirect (recurrent bronchial) connection of air sac to lung

FIGURE 3-26 Ventral View of the Avian Kidneys,
as well as Vessels and Nerves in their Vicinity

The right kidney shows the branches of the ureter, while the left kidney shows
the renal vessels. Cranial (*A*), middle (*B*), and caudal (*C*) divisions of kidney.

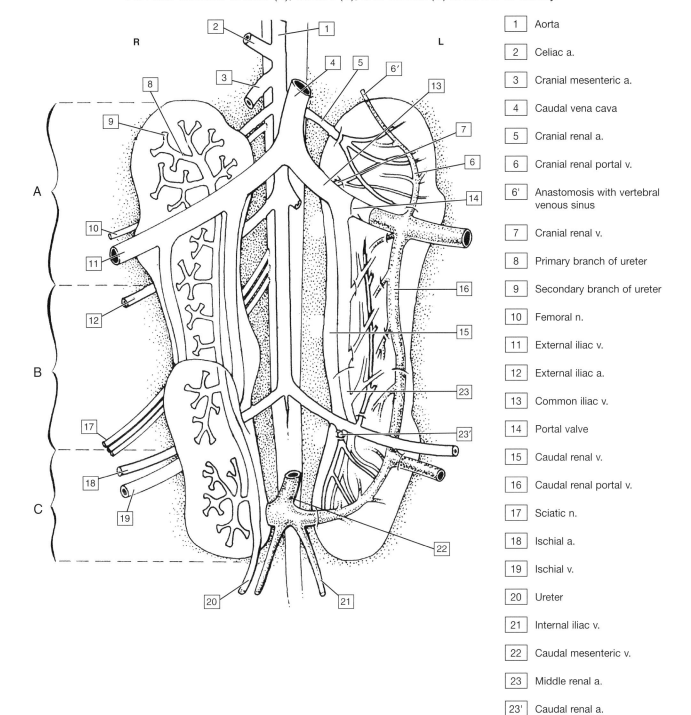

1	Aorta
2	Celiac a.
3	Cranial mesenteric a.
4	Caudal vena cava
5	Cranial renal a.
6	Cranial renal portal v.
6′	Anastomosis with vertebral venous sinus
7	Cranial renal v.
8	Primary branch of ureter
9	Secondary branch of ureter
10	Femoral n.
11	External iliac v.
12	External iliac a.
13	Common iliac v.
14	Portal valve
15	Caudal renal v.
16	Caudal renal portal v.
17	Sciatic n.
18	Ischial a.
19	Ischial v.
20	Ureter
21	Internal iliac v.
22	Caudal mesenteric v.
23	Middle renal a.
23′	Caudal renal a.

4 THE ABDOMEN

FIGURE 4-1   Schematic of the Digestive Apparatus

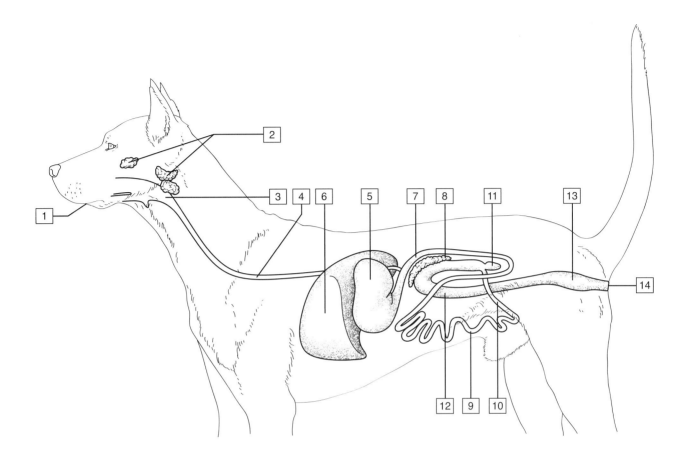

1	Mouth	5	Stomach	9	Jejunum	13	Rectum
2	Salivary glands	6	Liver	10	Ileum	14	Anus
3	Pharynx	7	Duodenum	11	Cecum		
4	Esophagus	8	Pancreas	12	Colon		

FIGURE 4-2 Rectus Sheath of the Canine in Transverse Sections

A, Cranial and *B,* caudal to the umbilicus and near the pubis, *C.*

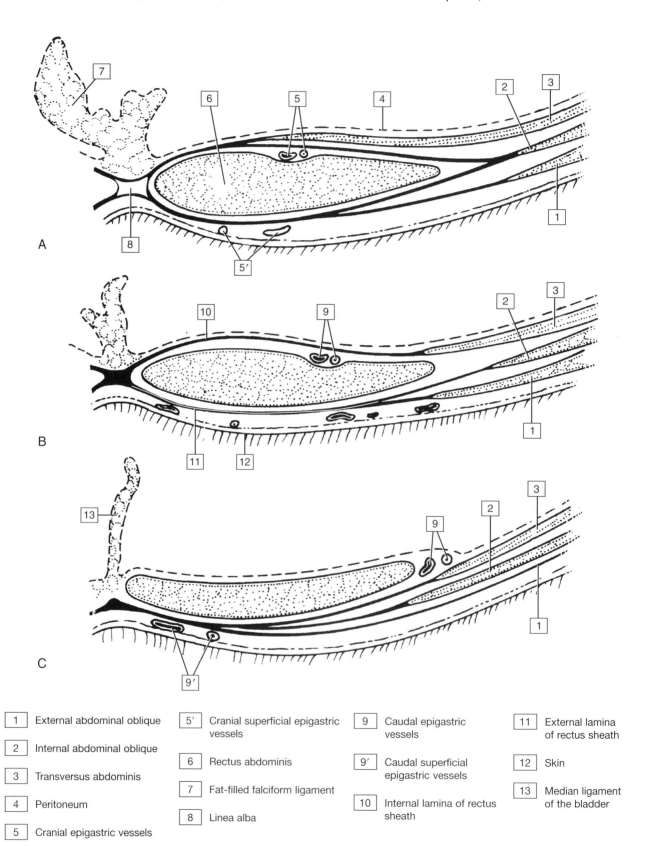

1	External abdominal oblique	5'	Cranial superficial epigastric vessels	9	Caudal epigastric vessels	11	External lamina of rectus sheath
2	Internal abdominal oblique						
3	Transversus abdominis	6	Rectus abdominis	9'	Caudal superficial epigastric vessels	12	Skin
4	Peritoneum	7	Fat-filled falciform ligament	10	Internal lamina of rectus sheath	13	Median ligament of the bladder
5	Cranial epigastric vessels	8	Linea alba				

FIGURE 4-3   Canine Inguinal Canal and Pelvic Diaphragm, Left Lateral View

The external abdominal oblique muscle has been removed.

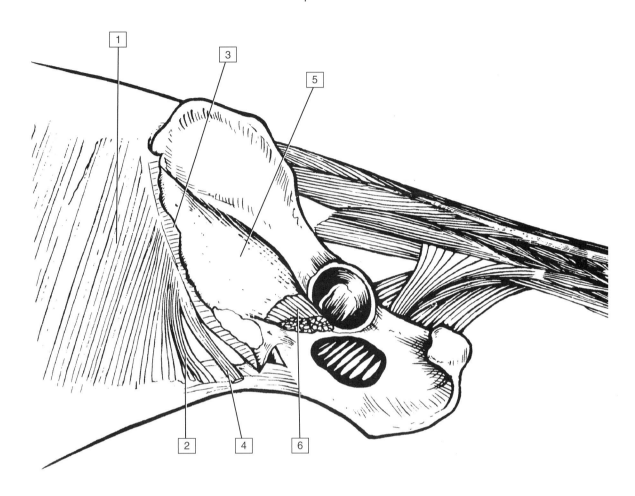

1	Internal abdominal oblique	4	Cremaster derived from internal oblique
2	Free caudal edge of internal oblique, forming border of deep inguinal ring	5	Iliac fascia covering iliopsoas
3	Stump of external oblique aponeurosis reflected caudally	6	Iliopsoas

FIGURE 4-4   Schematic Transverse Section Through the Canine Abdomen

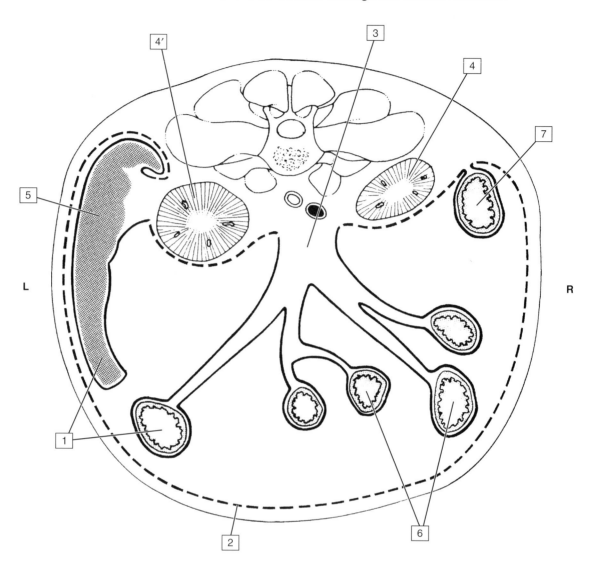

1	Visceral peritoneum (*continuous line*)	4′	Left kidney (retroperitoneal)
2	Parietal peritoneum (*broken line*)	5	Spleen
3	Root of mesentery	6	Jejunum
4	Right kidney (retroperitoneal)	7	Descending duodenum

Saunders Veterinary Anatomy Coloring Book

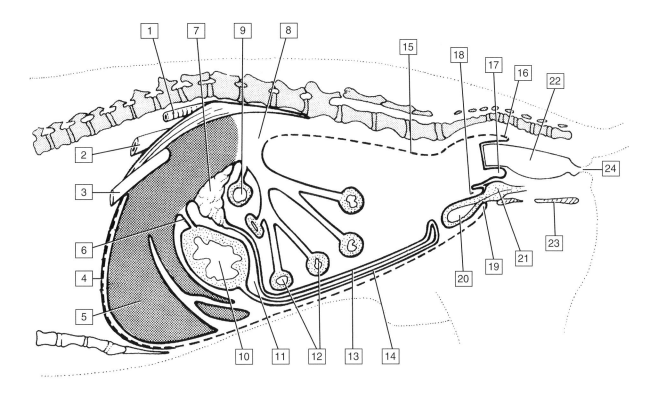

1	Aorta	13	Deep wall of greater omentum
2	Esophagus	14	Superficial wall of greater omentum
3	Caudal vena cava	15	Parietal peritoneum
4	Diaphragm	16	Pararectal fossa
5	Liver	17	Rectogenital pouch
6	Lesser omentum	18	Vesicogenital pouch
7	Pancreas	19	Pubovesical pouch
8	Root of mesentery	20	Bladder
9	Transverse colon	21	Prostate
10	Stomach	22	Rectum
11	Omental bursa	23	Ischium
12	Small intestine	24	Anus

FIGURE 4-6   Distribution of the Canine Celiac Artery, Ventral View

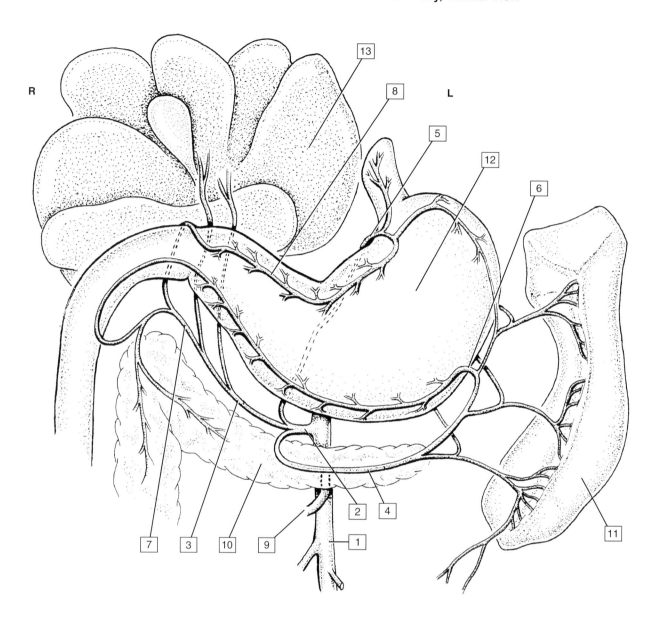

1	Aorta		8	Right gastric a.
2	Celiac a.		9	Cranial mesenteric a.
3	Hepatic a.		10	Pancreas
4	Splenic a.		11	Spleen
5	Left gastric a.		12	Stomach
6	Left gastroepiploic a.		13	Liver
7	Gastroduodenal a.			

FIGURE 4-7   Canine Abdominal Organs after
Removal of the Greater Omentum, Ventral View

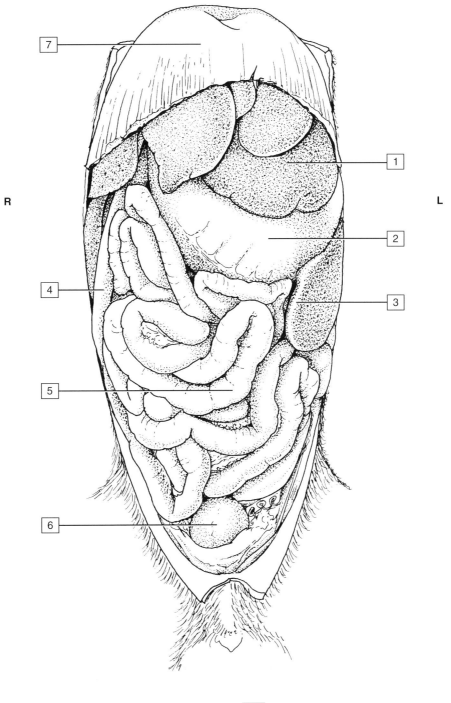

1	Liver	5	Jejunum
2	Stomach	6	Bladder
3	Spleen	7	Diaphragm
4	Descending duodenum		

FIGURE 4-8   Muscles of the Canine Perineal Region

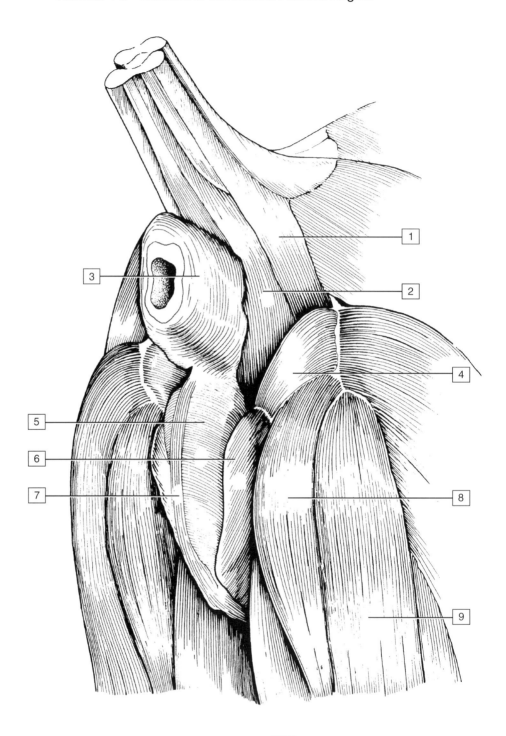

1	Coccygeus	6	Ischiocavernosus
2	Levator ani	7	Retractor penis
3	External anal sphincter	8	Semimembranosus
4	Internal obturator	9	Semitendinosus
5	Bulbospongiosus		

FIGURE 4-9 Distribution of the Canine Cranial and Caudal
Mesenteric Arteries to the Intestines, Dorsal View

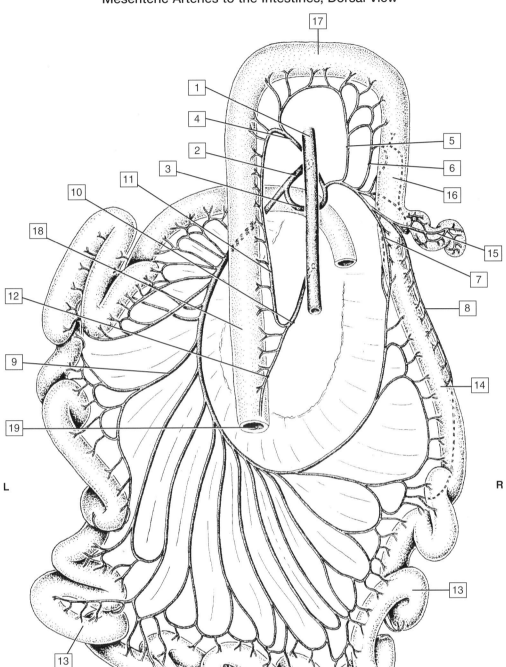

1	Aorta	6	Colic branch of ileocolic a.	11	Left colic a.	16	Ascending colon
2	Cranial mesenteric a.	7	Mesenteric ileal branch	12	Cranial rectal a.	17	Transverse colon
3	Ileocolic a.	8	Antimesenteric ileal branch	13	Jejunum	18	Descending colon
4	Middle colic a.	9	Jejunal aa.	14	Ileum	19	Rectum
5	Right colic a.	10	Caudal mesenteric a.	15	Cecum		

FIGURE 4-10   Semischematic Dorsal View
of the Formation of the Canine Portal Vein

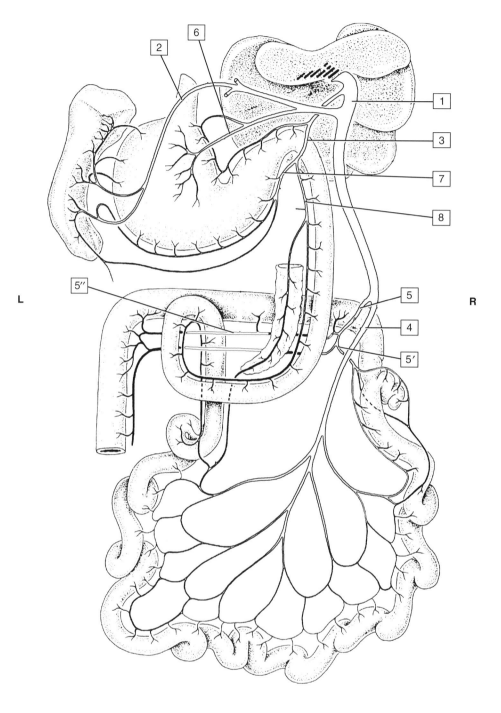

L   R

1	Portal vein	5′	Ileocolic vein
2	Splenic vein	5″	Middle colic vein
3	Gastroduodenal vein	6	Left gastric vein
4	Cranial mesenteric vein	7	Right gastroepiploic vein
5	Caudal mesenteric vein	8	Cranial pancreaticoduodenal vein

FIGURE 4-11   Visceral Surface of the Canine Liver

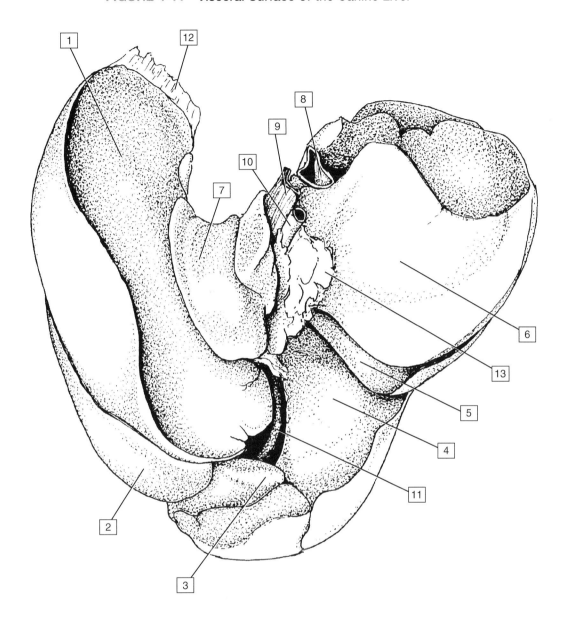

1	Left lateral lobe	8	Caudal vena cava
2	Left medial lobe	9	Portal vein
3	Quadrate lobe	10	Hepatic a.
4	Right medial lobe	11	Gallbladder
5	Right lateral lobe	12	Left triangular ligament
6	Caudate process (of caudate lobe)	13	Lesser omentum
7	Papillary process (of caudate lobe)		

FIGURE 4-12 Development of the Canine Liver

A, Early development: a cranial branch of the endodermal
diverticulum invades the septum transversum; a caudal branch forms
the gallbladder and cystic duct. *B,* A later stage, in which the developing
liver expands caudally into the abdominal cavity.

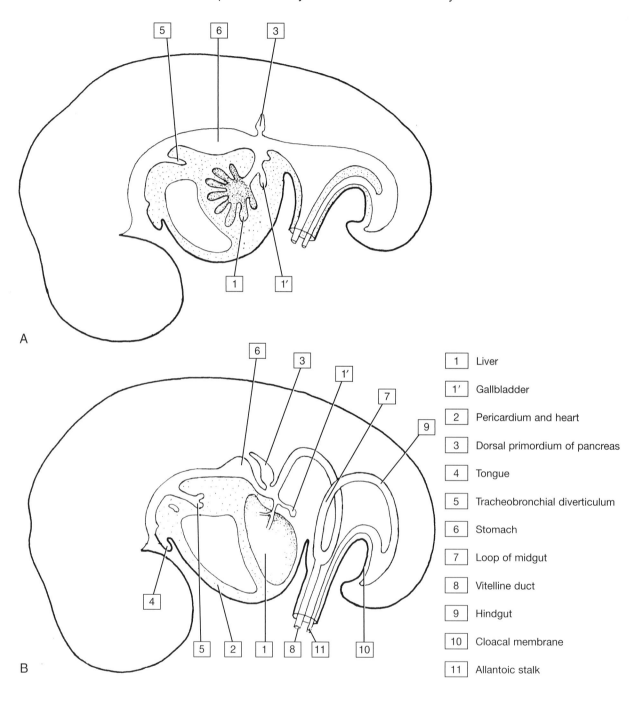

1 Liver
1′ Gallbladder
2 Pericardium and heart
3 Dorsal primordium of pancreas
4 Tongue
5 Tracheobronchial diverticulum
6 Stomach
7 Loop of midgut
8 Vitelline duct
9 Hindgut
10 Cloacal membrane
11 Allantoic stalk

FIGURE 4-13   Development of the Canine
Intestinal Tract during the Rotation Process

The midgut loop is herniated into the extraembryonic celom.

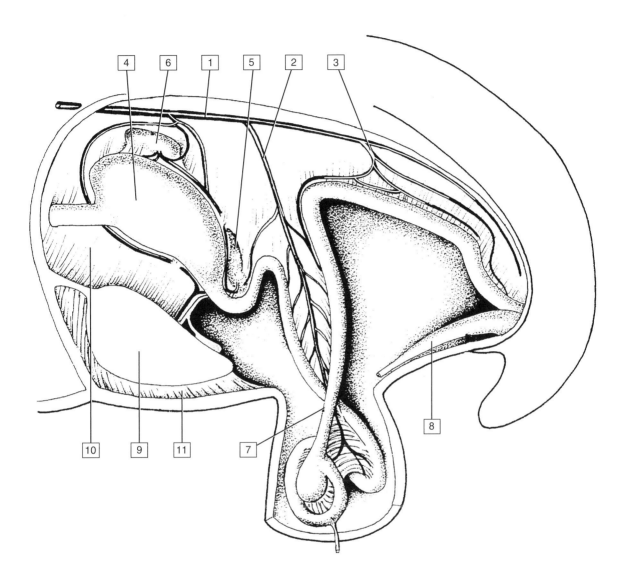

1	Celiac a.	7	Loop of midgut
2	Cranial mesenteric a.	8	Bladder expansion of the urogenital sinus
3	Caudal mesenteric a.	9	Liver
4	Stomach	10	Lesser omentum
5	Pancreas	11	Falciform ligament
6	Spleen		

FIGURE 4-14 Lymph Drainage from the Organs
in the Canine Abdominal and Pelvic Cavities

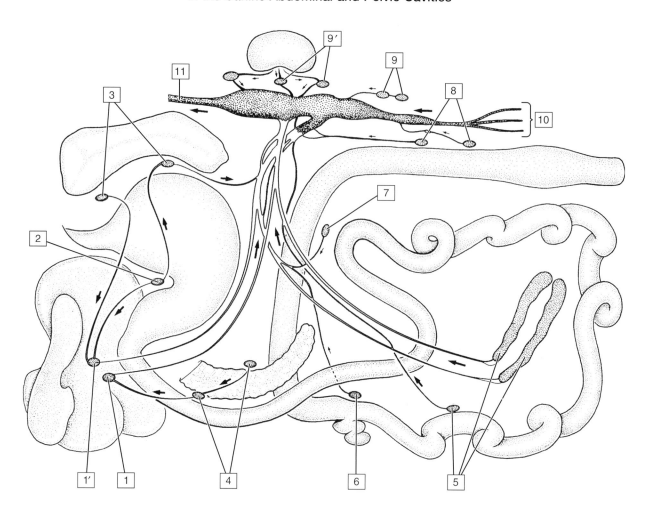

1	Right hepatic node	7	Middle colic node
1'	Left hepatic node	8	Caudal mesenteric nodes
2	Gastric node	9	Lumbar aortic nodes
3	Splenic nodes	9'	Renal nodes
4	Pancreaticoduodenal nodes	10	Efferents from the iliosacral region
5	Jejunal nodes	11	Continuation of cisterna chyli as thoracic duct
6	Right colic node		

FIGURE 4-15   Ganglia and Plexuses of the
Canine Abdominal Cavity, Ventral View

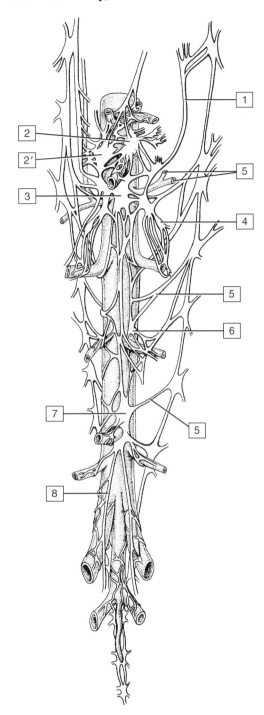

1	Greater splanchnic n.		5	Lumbar splanchnic n.
2	Left celiac ganglion		6	Gonadal ganglion
2′	Right celiac ganglion		7	Caudal mesenteric ganglion
3	Cranial mesenteric ganglion		8	Right hypogastric n.
4	Renal ganglion			

FIGURE 4-16   Transverse Section of the Canine
Trunk at the Level of the 11th Thoracic Vertebra

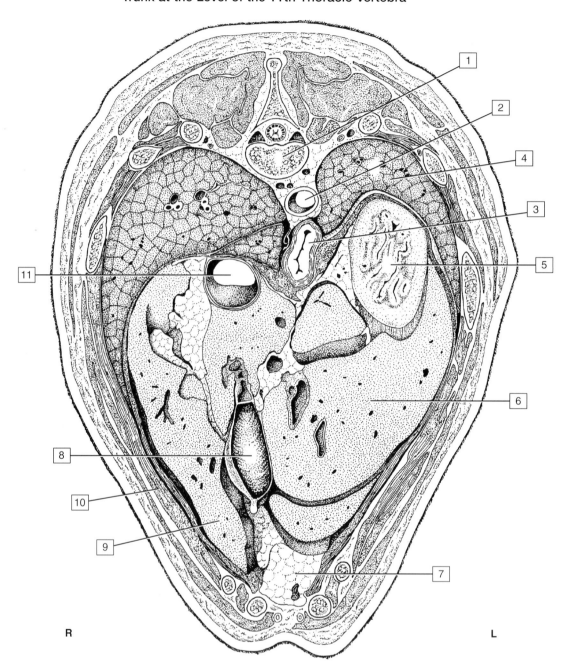

R   L

1	Eleventh thoracic vertebra	5	Fundus of stomach	9	Right medial lobe of liver
2	Aorta	6	Left lateral lobe of liver	10	Diaphragm
3	Esophagus	7	Fat-filled falciform ligament	11	Caudal vena cava
4	Left lung	8	Gallbladder		

FIGURE 4-17   Transverse Section of the Canine
Trunk at the Level of the 12th Thoracic Vertebra

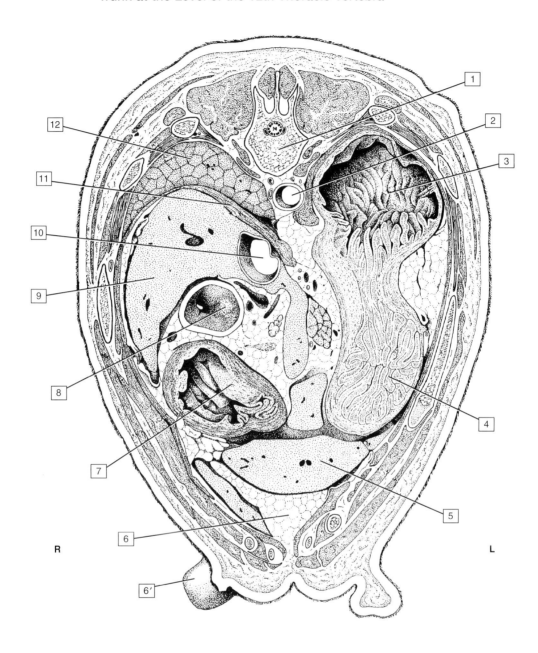

R   L

1	Twelfth thoracic vertebra	6	Fat-filled falciform ligament	10	Caudal vena cava
2	Aorta	6'	Teat	11	Diaphragm
3	Fundus of stomach	7	Pyloric part of stomach	12	Right lung
4	Body of stomach	8	Descending duodenum		
5	Liver	9	Caudate process of liver		

FIGURE 4-18   Transverse Sections of the Canine Abdomen at the Level
of the First Lumbar Vertebra (A) and Fourth or Fifth Lumbar Vertebra (B)

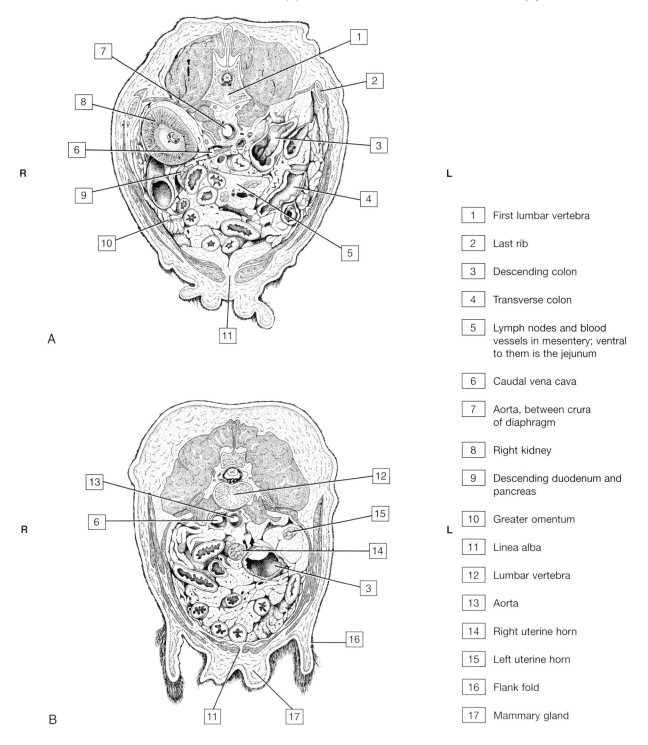

R

L

1	First lumbar vertebra
2	Last rib
3	Descending colon
4	Transverse colon
5	Lymph nodes and blood vessels in mesentery; ventral to them is the jejunum
6	Caudal vena cava
7	Aorta, between crura of diaphragm
8	Right kidney
9	Descending duodenum and pancreas
10	Greater omentum
11	Linea alba
12	Lumbar vertebra
13	Aorta
14	Right uterine horn
15	Left uterine horn
16	Flank fold
17	Mammary gland

FIGURE 4-19   The Blood Supply of the Canine Intestinal Tract, Ventral View

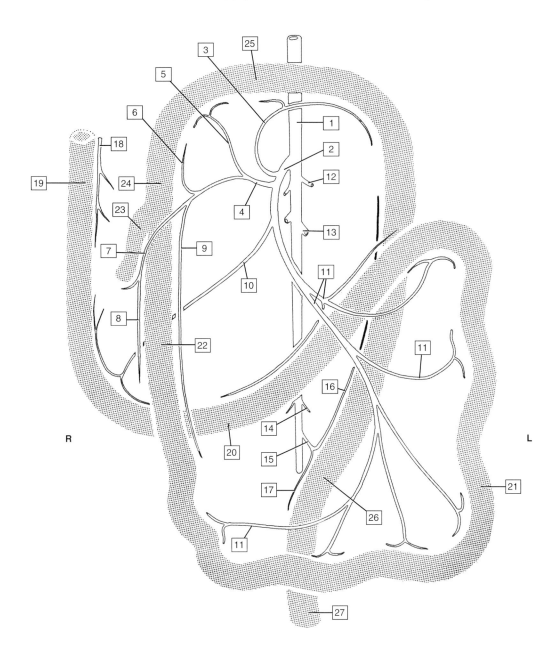

1	Abdominal aorta	8	Antimesenteric ileal branch	14	Testicular (ovarian) aa.	21	Jejunum
2	Cranial mesenteric a.	9	Mesenteric ileal branch	15	Caudal mesenteric aa.	22	Ileum
3	Middle colic a.	10	Caudal pancreaticoduodenal a.	16	Left colic a.	23	Cecum
4	Ileocolic a.	11	Jejunal aa.	17	Cranial rectal a.	24	Ascending colon
5	Right colic a.	12	Phrenicoabdominal aa.	18	Cranial pancreaticoduodenal a.	25	Transverse colon
6	Colic branch of ileocolic a.	13	Renal a.	19	Descending duodenum	26	Descending colon
7	Cecal a.			20	Ascending duodenum	27	Rectum

FIGURE 4-20 Canine Abdominal Muscles and
Inguinal Region of the Male, Deep Dissection, Left Side

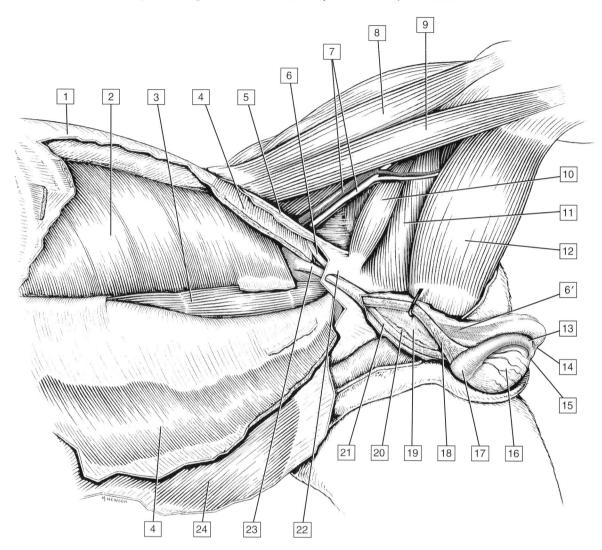

1 Thoracolumbar fascia	8 Cranial part of sartorius	18 Testicular artery and vein in visceral vaginal tunic (mesorchium)
2 Transversus abdominis	9 Caudal part of sartorius	19 Mesorchium
3 Rectus abdominis	10 Pectineus	20 Mesoductus deferens
4 Internal abdominal oblique (transected and reflected)	11 Adductor	21 Ductus deferens in visceral vaginal tunic
5 Inguinal ligament (caudal border of aponeurosis of external abdominal oblique muscle)	12 Gracilis	22 Superficial inguinal ring, lateral crus
	13 Tail of epididymis	23 Parietal vaginal tunic in the inguinal canal
6 Cremaster muscle at its origin	14 Ligament of tail of epididymis	
6′ Cremaster muscle on external surface of parietal layer of vaginal tunic	15 Proper ligament of testis	24 External abdominal oblique (reflected)
	16 Testis in visceral vaginal tunic	
7 Femoral artery and vein	17 Head of epididymis	

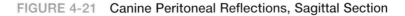

FIGURE 4-21 Canine Peritoneal Reflections, Sagittal Section

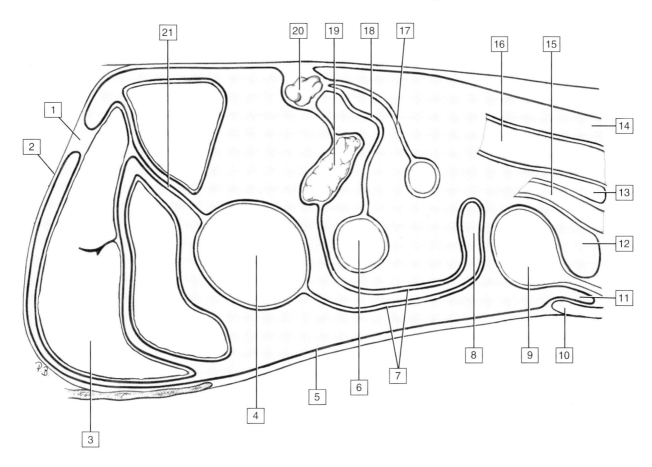

1	Coronary ligament		12	Vesicogenital pouch
2	Diaphragm		13	Rectogenital pouch
3	Liver		14	Pararectal fossa
4	Stomach		15	Uterus
5	Parietal peritoneum		16	Descending colon
6	Transverse colon		17	Mesentery
7	Greater omentum, deep and superficial leaves		18	Transverse mesocolon
8	Omental bursa		19	Left lobe, pancreas
9	Bladder		20	Lymph nodes
10	Symphysis		21	Lesser omentum
11	Pubovesical pouch			

FIGURE 4-22   Canine Liver, Visceral Aspect

Dog in dorsal recumbency, caudal to cranial view.

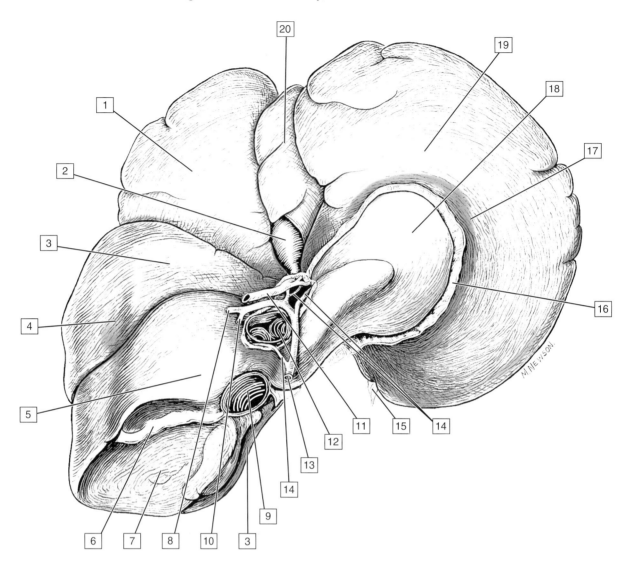

1	Right medial lobe	8	Gastroduodenal artery	15	Left triangular ligament
2	Gallbladder	9	Right lateral lobe	16	Lesser omentum
3	Right lateral lobe	10	Right gastric artery	17	Gastric impression
4	Duodenal impression	11	Bile duct	18	Papillary process of caudate lobe
5	Caudate process of caudate lobe	12	Portal vein	19	Left lateral lobe
6	Hepatorenal ligament	13	Hepatic artery	20	Caudate lobe
7	Renal fossa	14	Hepatic branches		

Saunders Veterinary Anatomy Coloring Book

FIGURE 4-23 Canine Branches of Celiac and Cranial
Mesenteric Arteries with Principal Anastomoses

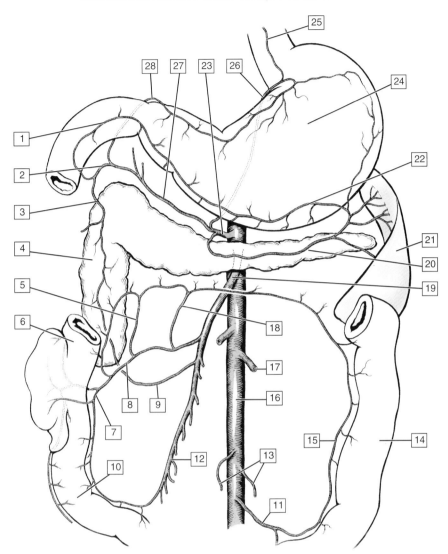

1	Right gastroepiploic a.	8	Ileocolic a.	15	Left colic a.	22	Left gastroepiploic a.
2	Gastroduodenal a.	9	Caudal pancreaticoduodenal a.	16	Aorta a.	23	Celiac a.
3	Cranial pancreaticoduodenal a.	10	Ileum	17	Left renal a.	24	Stomach
4	Pancreas	11	Caudal mesenteric a.	18	Middle colic a.	25	Esophageal a.
5	Right colic a.	12	Jejunal aa.	19	Cranial mesenteric a.	26	Left gastric a.
6	Ascending colon	13	Testucular (ovarian) aa.	20	Splenic a.	27	Hepatic a.
7	Cecal a.	14	Descending colon	21	Spleen	28	Right gastric a.

Is this the dorsal or ventral view?

Saunders Veterinary Anatomy Coloring Book

FIGURE 4-24   The Attachment of the Equine Abdominal
Muscles on the Pelvis and the Prepubic Tendon

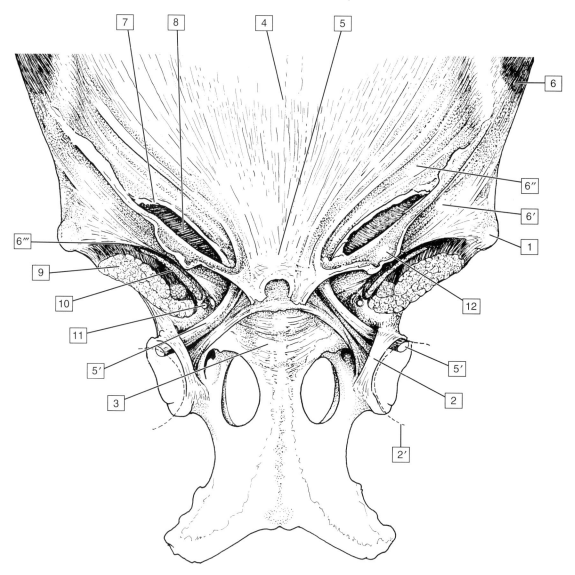

1	Coxal tuber	6''	Pelvic tendon of external oblique aponeurosis
2	Transverse acetabular ligament	6'''	Attachment of pelvic tendon of external oblique aponeurosis on sartorius and iliopsoas ("inguinal ligament")
2'	Femoral head		
3	Pubis	7	Superficial inguinal ring
4	Tunica flava over linea alba	8	Internal abdominal oblique
5	Prepubic tendon	9	Iliopsoas
5'	Accessory ligament	10	Sartorius
6	External abdominal oblique	11	Vascular lacuna containing femoral vessels
6'	Pelvic tendon of external oblique	12	Femoral fascia (lamina)

FIGURE 4-25 Equine Abdominal Muscles and their Skeletal Attachments

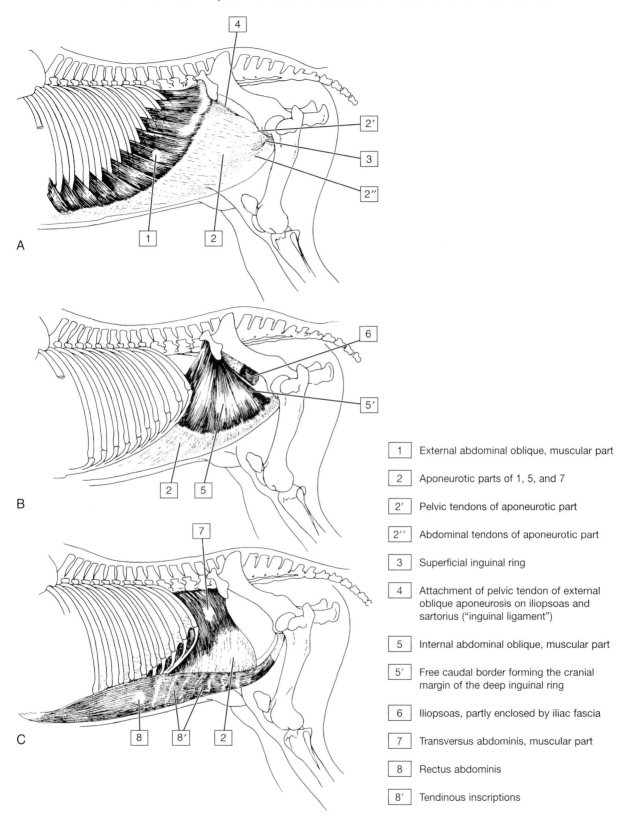

1	External abdominal oblique, muscular part
2	Aponeurotic parts of 1, 5, and 7
2′	Pelvic tendons of aponeurotic part
2″	Abdominal tendons of aponeurotic part
3	Superficial inguinal ring
4	Attachment of pelvic tendon of external oblique aponeurosis on iliopsoas and sartorius ("inguinal ligament")
5	Internal abdominal oblique, muscular part
5′	Free caudal border forming the cranial margin of the deep inguinal ring
6	Iliopsoas, partly enclosed by iliac fascia
7	Transversus abdominis, muscular part
8	Rectus abdominis
8′	Tendinous inscriptions

FIGURE 4-26 Visceral Surface of the Equine Spleen

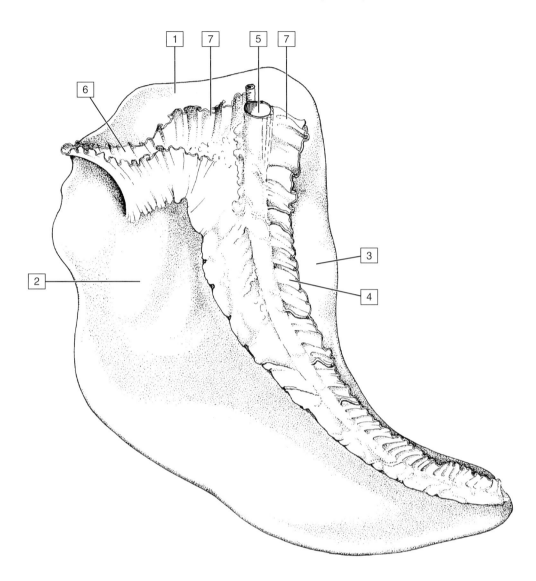

1	Renal surface	5	Splenic artery and vein
2	Intestinal surface	6	Renosplenic ligament
3	Gastric surface	7	Phrenicosplenic ligament
4	Greater omentum (gastrosplenic ligament)		

Saunders Veterinary Anatomy Coloring Book

FIGURE 4-27   Interior of the Equine
Stomach and Cranial Part of the Duodenum

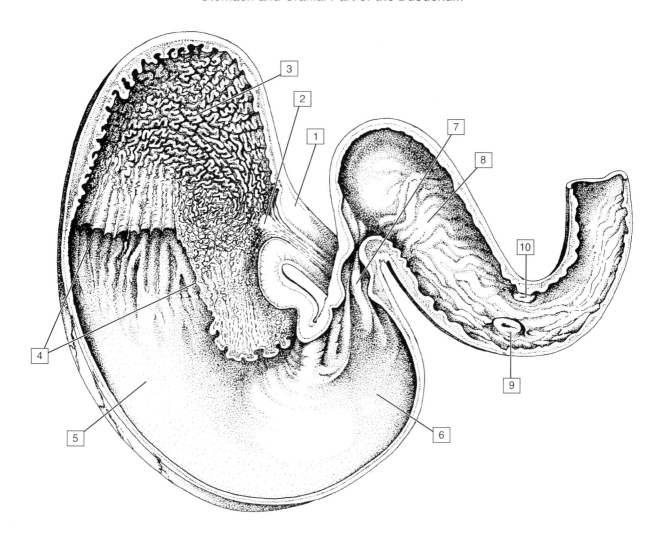

1	Esophagus	6	Pyloric part
2	Cardiac opening	7	Pylorus
3	Fundus (blind sac)	8	Cranial part of duodenum
4	Margo plicatus	9	Major duodenal papilla within hepatopancreatic ampulla
5	Body	10	Minor duodenal papilla

FIGURE 4-28   Equine Intestinal Tract Seen from the Right

The caudal flexure of the duodenum and the cranial mesenteric artery have been displaced to the right of the animal to lie over the base of the cecum.

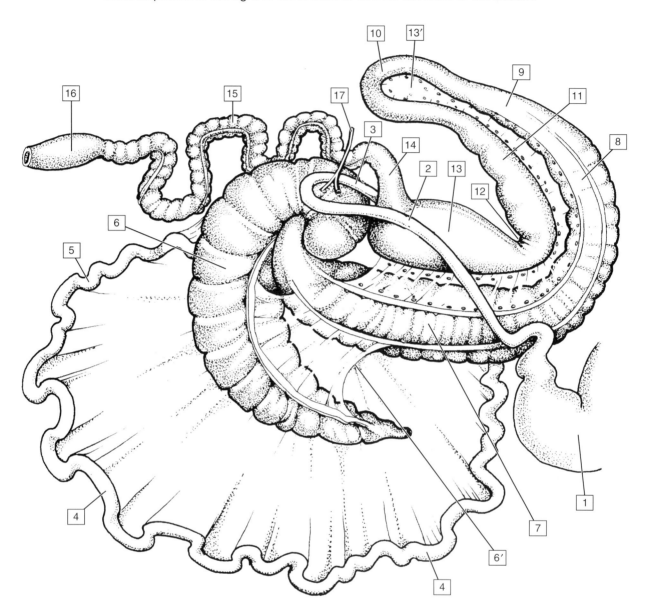

1	Stomach	7	Right ventral colon	13′	Ascending mesocolon
2	Descending duodenum	8	Ventral diaphragmatic flexure	14	Transverse colon
3	Ascending duodenum	9	Left ventral colon	15	Descending (small) colon
4	Jejunum	10	Pelvic flexure	16	Rectum
5	Ileum	11	Left dorsal colon	17	Cranial mesenteric artery
6	Cecum	12	Dorsal diaphragmatic flexure		
6′	Cecocolic fold	13	Right dorsal colon		

FIGURE 4-29   Position of the Equine Large
Intestine and the Kidneys, Dorsal View

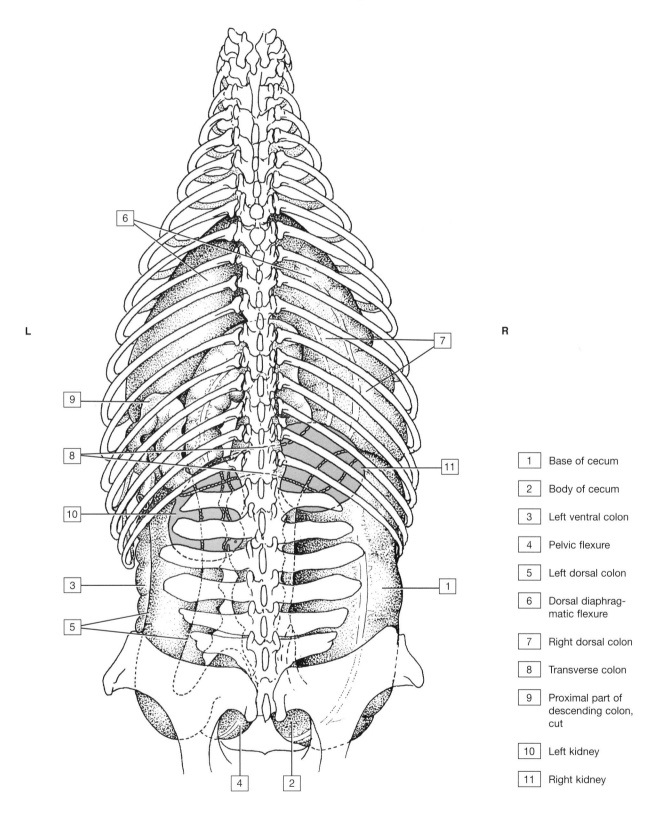

L

R

1	Base of cecum
2	Body of cecum
3	Left ventral colon
4	Pelvic flexure
5	Left dorsal colon
6	Dorsal diaphrag-matic flexure
7	Right dorsal colon
8	Transverse colon
9	Proximal part of descending colon, cut
10	Left kidney
11	Right kidney

FIGURE 4-30   Topography of the Equine Spleen,
Stomach, Pancreas, and Liver, Caudoventral View

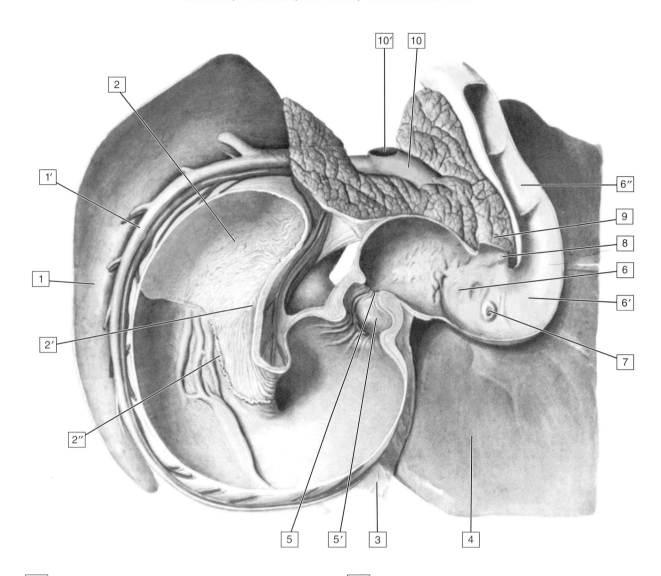

1	Intestinal surface of spleen	6	S-shaped cranial part of duodenum
1'	Splenic a. and v.	6'	Cranial flexure of duodenum
2	Fundus (blind sac) of stomach	6''	Descending duodenum
2'	Cardia	7	Major duodenal papilla
2''	Margo plicatus	8	Minor duodenal papilla
3	Greater omentum	9	Body of pancreas
4	Liver	10	Portal v.
5	Pyloric orifice	10'	Stump of cranial mesenteric v.
5'	Pyloric antrum		

FIGURE 4-31

Relationship of the lumbar spinal nerves to the
transverse processes of the bovine lumbar vertebrae

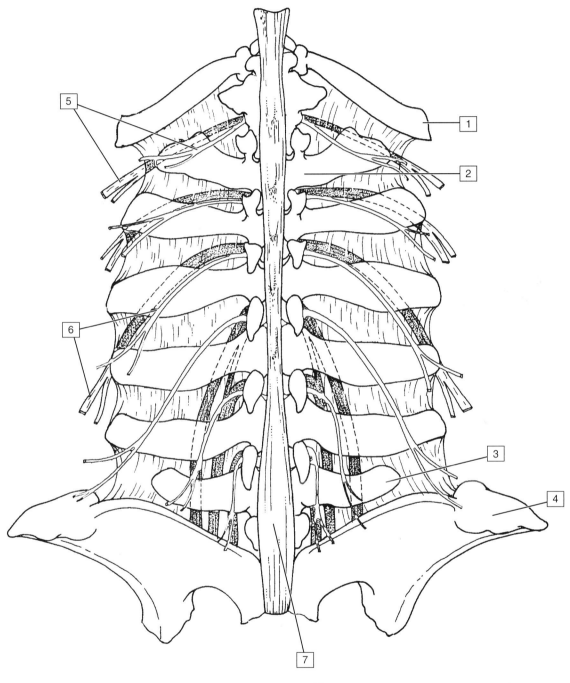

1	Last rib	5	Dorsal and ventral branches of 13th thoracic nerve (the ventral branch is partly stippled)
2	First lumbar vertebra	6	Dorsal and ventral branches of second lumbar nerve
3	Sixth lumbar vertebra	7	Supraspinous ligament
4	Coxal tuber		

FIGURE 4-32 Topography of the Bovine Abdominal Viscera

A, Relationship of abdominal viscera to the left abdominal wall. *B*, Relationship of abdominal viscera to the right abdominal wall; the liver has been removed.

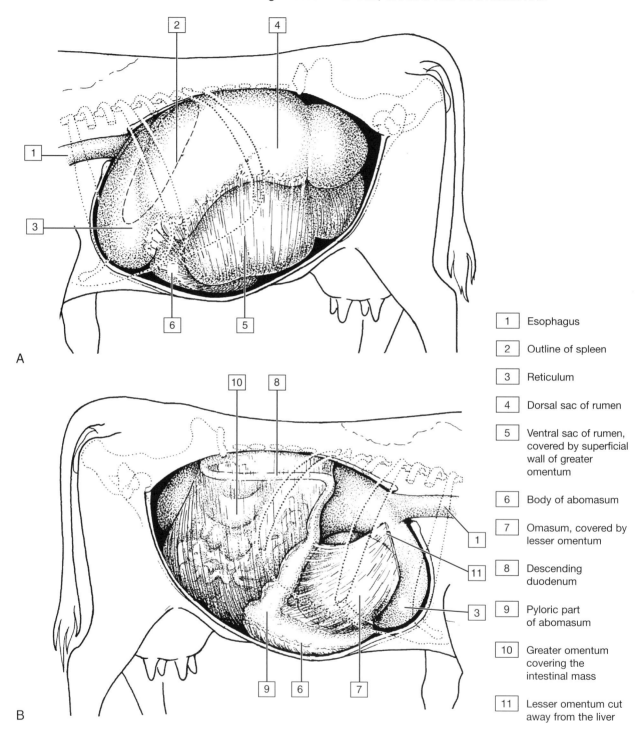

1	Esophagus
2	Outline of spleen
3	Reticulum
4	Dorsal sac of rumen
5	Ventral sac of rumen, covered by superficial wall of greater omentum
6	Body of abomasum
7	Omasum, covered by lesser omentum
8	Descending duodenum
9	Pyloric part of abomasum
10	Greater omentum covering the intestinal mass
11	Lesser omentum cut away from the liver

A

B

FIGURE 4-33

Bovine greater omentum fenestrated to permit
a view into omental bursa, caudal view

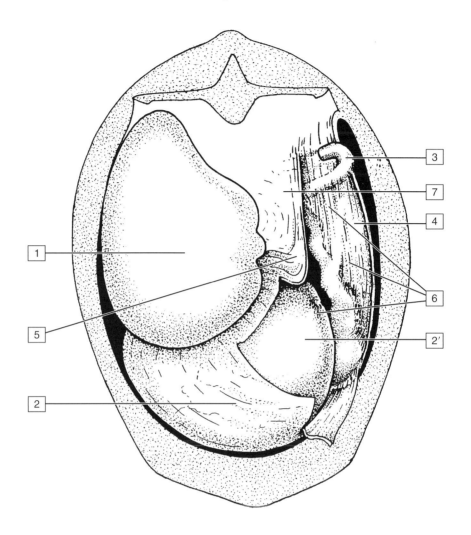

1	Dorsal sac of rumen		4	Superficial wall of greater omentum
2	Ventral sac of rumen, covered by superficial wall of greater omentum		5	Deep wall of greater omentum
2′	Ventral sac of rumen projecting into omental bursa		6	Omental bursa
3	Caudal flexure of duodenum		7	Supraomental recess

FIGURE 4-34   Right Lateral View of the Bovine Intestinal Tract

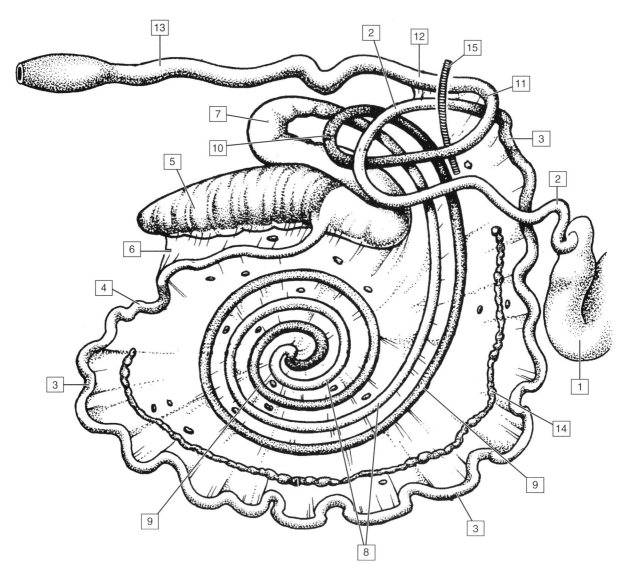

1	Pyloric part of abomasum	8	Centripetal turns of spiral colon
2	Duodenum	9	Centrifugal turns of spiral colon
3	Jejunum	10	Distal loop of ascending colon
4	Ileum	11	Transverse colon
5	Cecum	12	Descending colon
6	Ileocecal fold	13	Rectum

7–10 Ascending colon:

7	Proximal loop of ascending colon	14	Jejunal lymph nodes
		15	Cranial mesenteric a.

FIGURE 4-35

Permanent dentition of cattle, upper (*A*) and lower (*B*) jaws

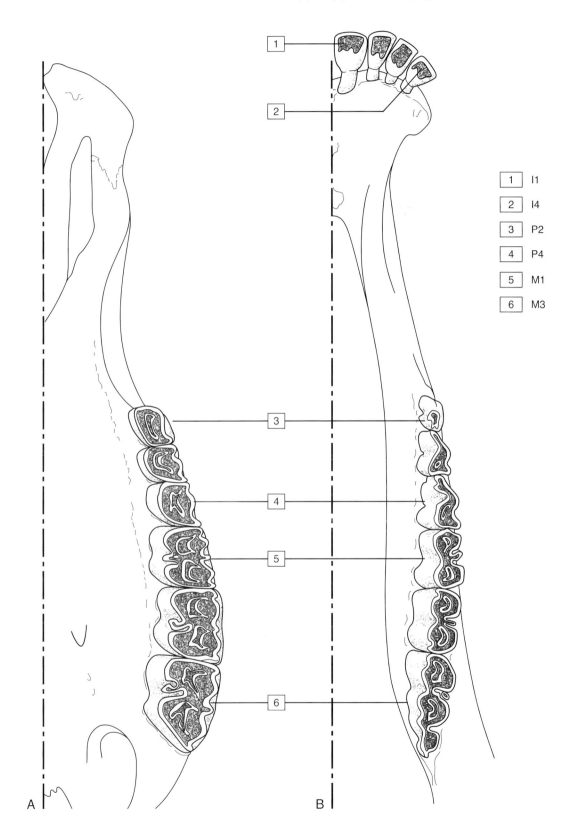

1	I1
2	I4
3	P2
4	P4
5	M1
6	M3

FIGURE 4-36   Male Porcine Inguinal Canal, Cranial View

Made visible on the interior (deep) surface of the caudal abdominal wall

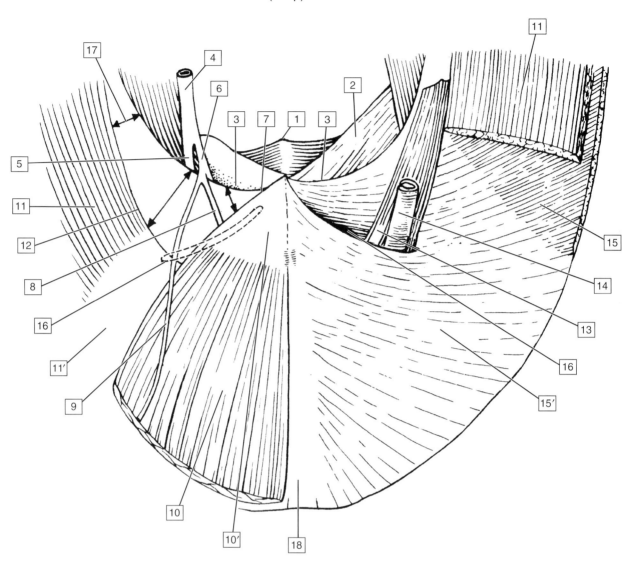

1	Pelvic symphysis	9	Caudal epigastric a.	14	Tunica vaginalis and spermatic cord
2	Prepubic tendon	10	Rectus abdominis	15	Muscular part of external abdominal oblique
3	Caudal border of external oblique aponeurosis ("inguinal ligament")	10'	Rectus tendon	15'	Aponeurotic part of external abdominal oblique
4	External iliac a.	11	Muscular part of internal abdominal oblique	16	Superficial inguinal ring
5	Femoral a.	11'	Aponeurotic part of internal abdominal oblique	17	Deep inguinal ring (*arrows*)
6	Deep femoral a.	12	Caudal free border of internal abdominal oblique	18	Linea alba
7	Lateral border of rectus tendon	13	Cremaster		
8	External pudendal a.				

FIGURE 4-37   Development of the Porcine Ascending Colon, Left Lateral View

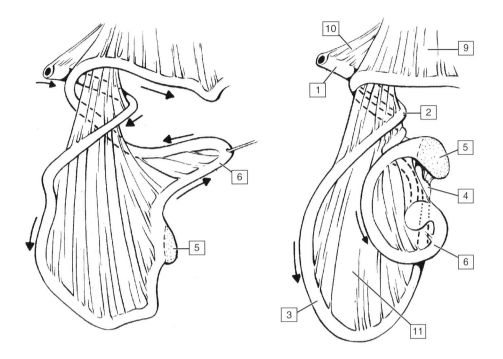

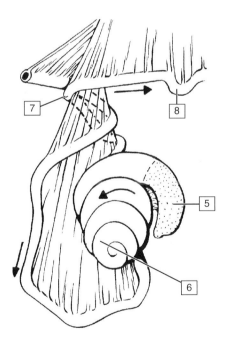

1	Descending duodenum
2	Caudal flexure of duodenum
3	Jejunum
4	Ileum
5	Cecum
6	Ascending colon
7	Transverse colon
8	Descending colon
9	Descending mesocolon
10	Mesoduodenum
11	Mesentery

FIGURE 4-38   Major Porcine Abdominal Arteries and Lymph Nodes

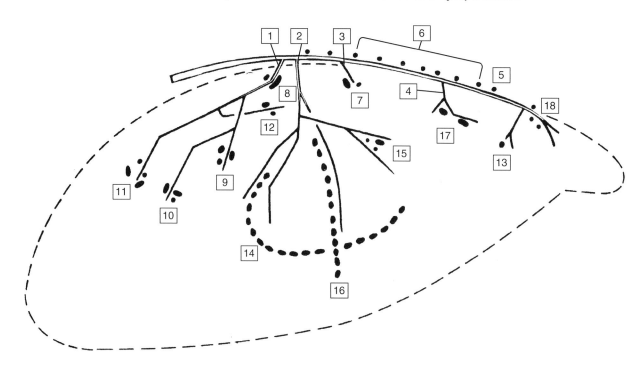

1 Celiac a.	10 Gastric nodes
2 Cranial mesenteric a.	11 Hepatic nodes
3 Renal a.	12 Pancreaticoduodenal nodes
4 Caudal mesenteric a.	13 Lateral iliac nodes
5 Deep circumflex iliac a.	14 Jejunal nodes
6 Lumbar aortic nodes	15 Ileocolic nodes
7 Renal nodes	16 Colic nodes
8 Celiac nodes	17 Caudal mesenteric nodes
9 Splenic nodes	18 Medial iliac nodes

FIGURE 4-39

Permanent dentition of the pig, upper (*A*) and lower (*B*) jaws

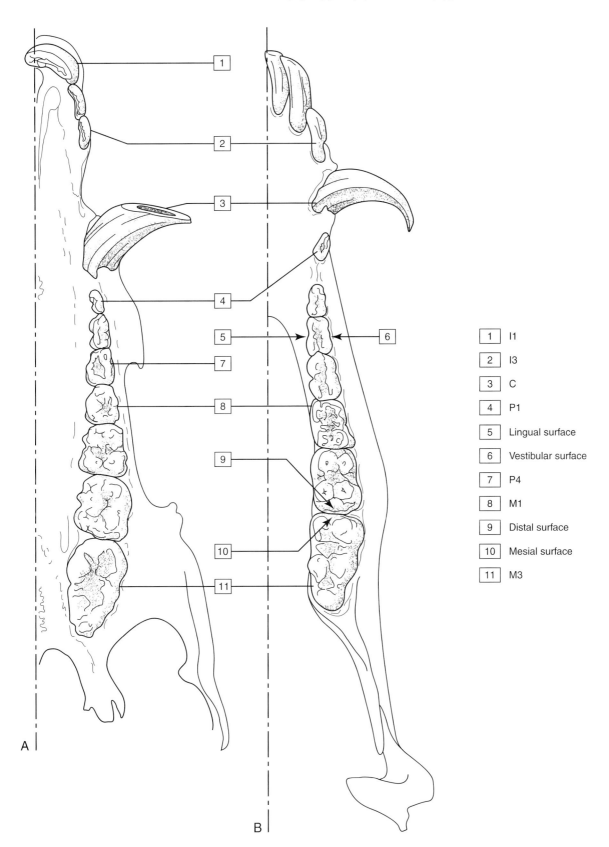

1	I1
2	I3
3	C
4	P1
5	Lingual surface
6	Vestibular surface
7	P4
8	M1
9	Distal surface
10	Mesial surface
11	M3

FIGURE 4-40

Avian gastrointestinal tract after reflection of liver,
stomach, and small intestine craniodextrally, ventral view

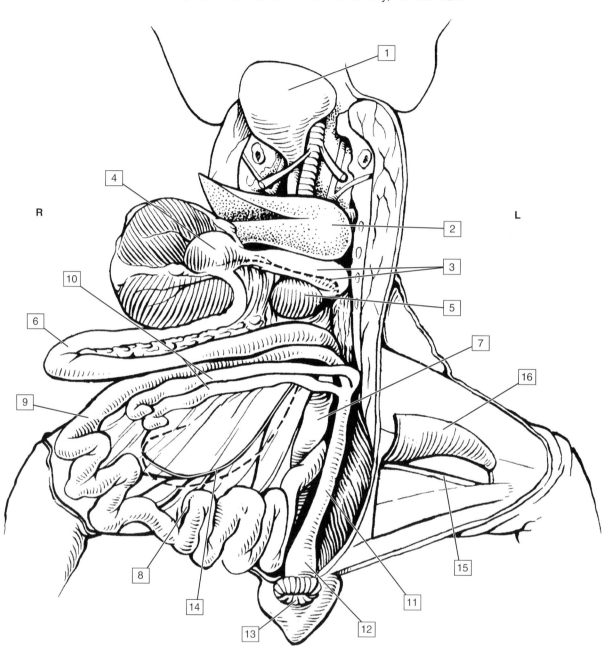

1 Crop	**6** Duodenal loop enclosing pancreas	**12** Cloaca
2 Left lobe of liver	**7** Jejunum	**13** Vent
3 Proventriculus with vagus on dorsal surface	**8** Vitelline diverticulum	**14** Cranial mesenteric vessels and intestinal nerve in mesentery
4 Cranial blind sac on right side of reflected gizzard	**9** Ileum	**15** Sciatic nerve and ischial a.
	10 Ceca	
5 Spleen	**11** Colon	**16** Gracilis and adductor

FIGURE 4-41

Canine, equine, and bovine
gastrointestinal tracts laid out in one plane

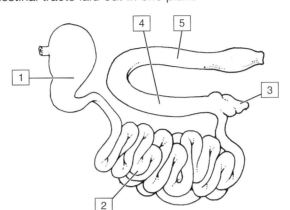

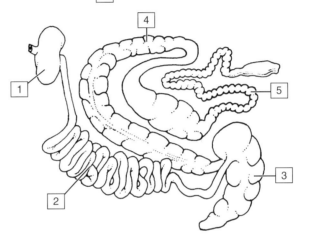

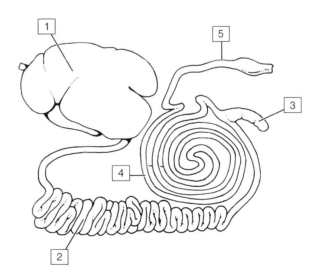

1	Stomach	4	Ascending colon
2	Small intestine	5	Descending colon
3	Cecum		

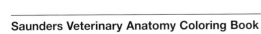

FIGURE 4-42

Canine and feline (*A*), porcine (*B*),
bovine (*C*), and equine (*D*) large intestine
Cranial is to the upper right

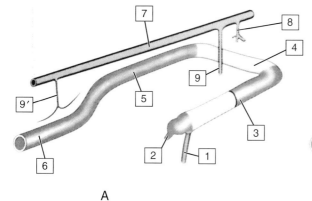

A

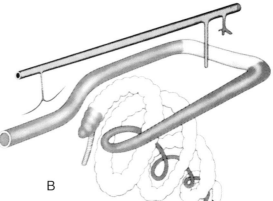

B

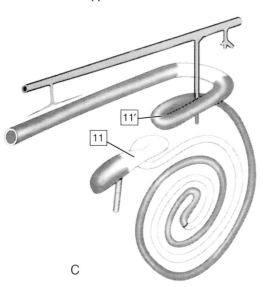

C

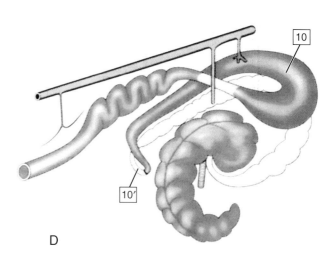

D

1	Ileum	8	Celiac a.
2	Cecum	9	Cranial mesenteric a.
3	Ascending colon	9′	Caudal mesenteric a.
4	Transverse colon	10	Dorsal diaphragmatic flexures of ascending colon
5	Descending colon	10′	Pelvic flexures of ascending colon
6	Rectum and anus	11	Proximal loop of ascending colon
7	Aorta	11′	Distal loop of ascending colon

FIGURE 4-43

Transverse section through the gut (general anatomy)

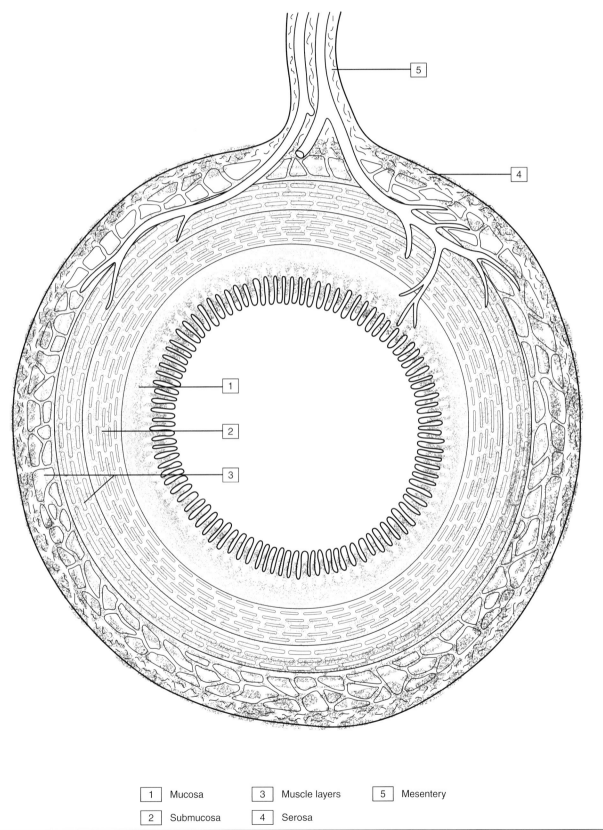

| 1 | Mucosa | 3 | Muscle layers | 5 | Mesentery |
| 2 | Submucosa | 4 | Serosa | | |

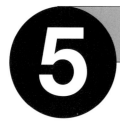

THE PELVIS AND REPRODUCTIVE ORGANS

FIGURE 5-1   Canine Sacrum, Cranial View

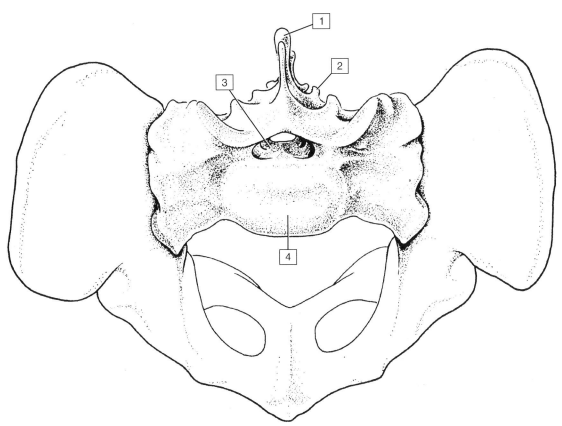

| 1 | Spinous process | 3 | Vertebral canal |
| 2 | Rudimentary articular process | 4 | Body |

FIGURE 5-2   Sagittal Section of an Early Canine Embryo

Part of the yolk sac is taken into the body in the folding process.

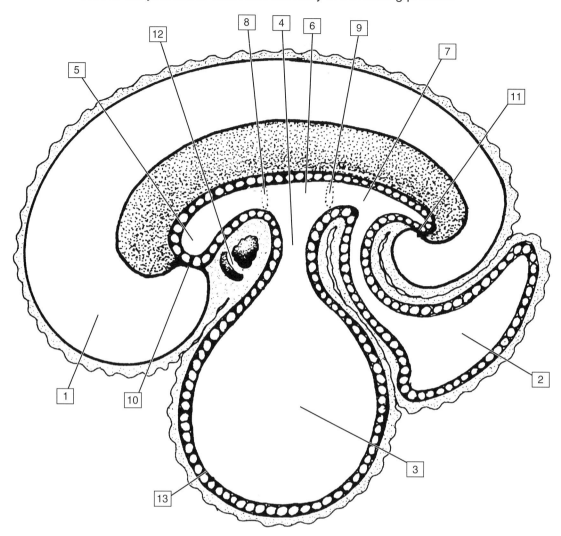

1	Amniotic cavity	8	Cranial intestinal portal
2	Allantoic cavity	9	Caudal intestinal portal
3	Yolk sac	10	Oral plate
4	Stalk of yolk sac	11	Cloacal plate
5	Foregut	12	Heart and pericardial cavity
6	Midgut	13	Endoderm
7	Hindgut		

THE PELVIS AND REPRODUCTIVE ORGANS 5

FIGURE 5-3 Canine Urinary and Male and Female Reproductive Organs

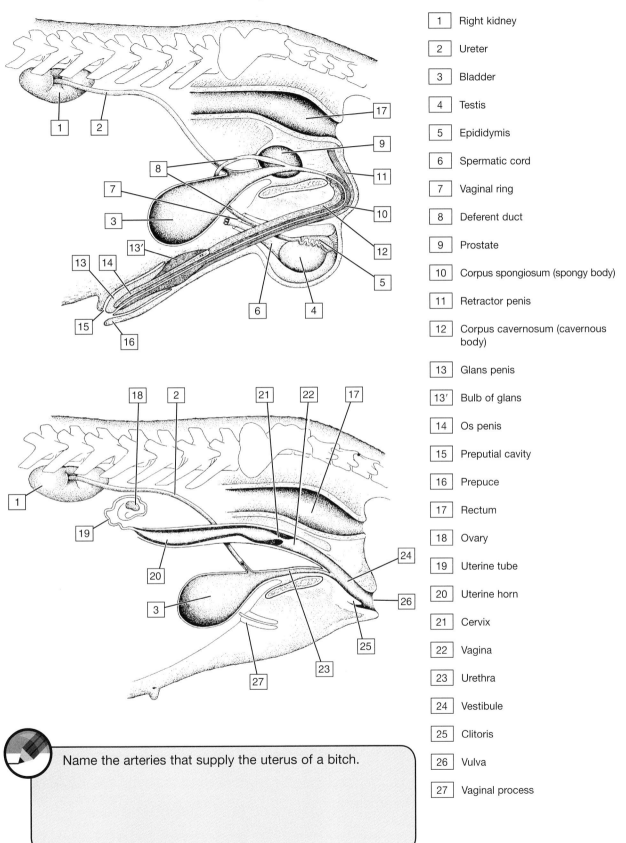

1	Right kidney
2	Ureter
3	Bladder
4	Testis
5	Epididymis
6	Spermatic cord
7	Vaginal ring
8	Deferent duct
9	Prostate
10	Corpus spongiosum (spongy body)
11	Retractor penis
12	Corpus cavernosum (cavernous body)
13	Glans penis
13'	Bulb of glans
14	Os penis
15	Preputial cavity
16	Prepuce
17	Rectum
18	Ovary
19	Uterine tube
20	Uterine horn
21	Cervix
22	Vagina
23	Urethra
24	Vestibule
25	Clitoris
26	Vulva
27	Vaginal process

Name the arteries that supply the uterus of a bitch.

FIGURE 5-4   Three Stages in the Development of the Canine Testis

A, The epithelial cords are isolated from the surface epithelium by the formation of the tunica albuginea. *B,* The epithelial cords, rete, and mesonephric tubules have interconnected. *C,* The epithelial cords become seminiferous tubules, and the mesonephros is gradually transformed into part of the epididymis.

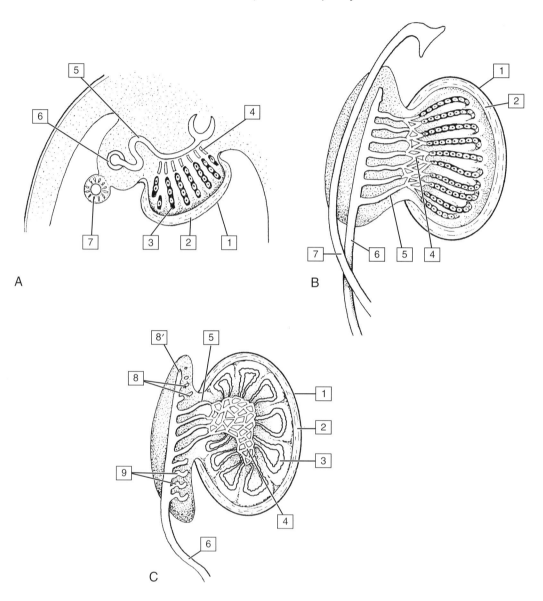

1	Celom epithelium	6	Mesonephric (later deferent) duct
2	Tunica albuginea	7	Paramesonephric duct
3	Epithelial cords, seminiferous tubules	8	Cranial remnant of mesonephric tubules (aberrant ductules)
4	Rete testis	8′	Remnant of 6 (appendix of epididymis)
5	Mesonephric tubules, efferent ductules	9	Caudal remnant (paradidymis)

FIGURE 5-5   Canine Kidney Lobe

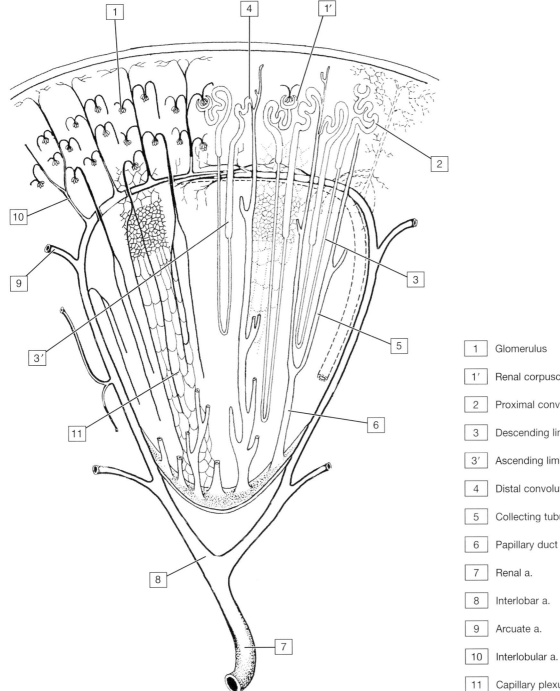

1	Glomerulus
1'	Renal corpuscle
2	Proximal convoluted tubule
3	Descending limb of nephron
3'	Ascending limb
4	Distal convoluted tubule
5	Collecting tubule
6	Papillary duct
7	Renal a.
8	Interlobar a.
9	Arcuate a.
10	Interlobular a.
11	Capillary plexus

FIGURE 5-6 Longitudinal Section of Canine Testis and Epididymis

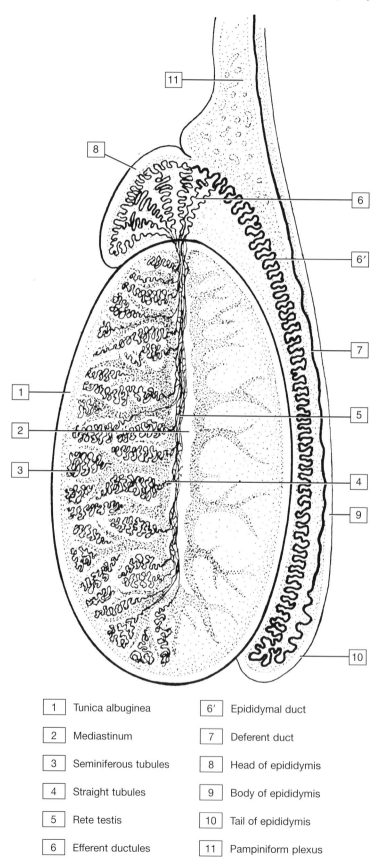

1	Tunica albuginea	6′	Epididymal duct
2	Mediastinum	7	Deferent duct
3	Seminiferous tubules	8	Head of epididymis
4	Straight tubules	9	Body of epididymis
5	Rete testis	10	Tail of epididymis
6	Efferent ductules	11	Pampiniform plexus

Saunders Veterinary Anatomy Coloring Book

FIGURE 5-7   Different Functional Stages in Canine Ovarian Activity

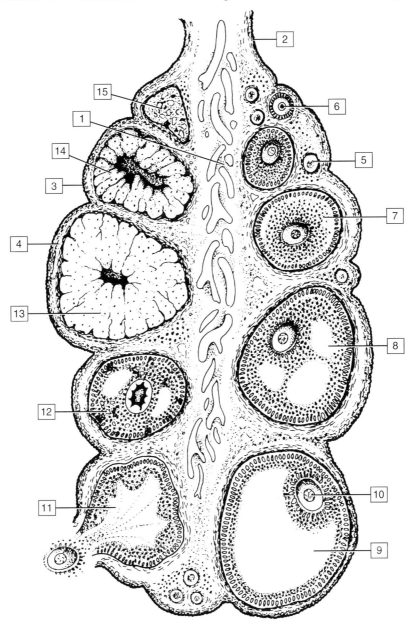

1	Medulla	5	Primordial follicle
2	Mesovarium	6	Primary follicle
3	Surface epithelium	7	Secondary follicle
4	Tunica albuginea (poorly developed)	8	Early tertiary follicle

9	Mature follicle	13	Corpus luteum
10	Oocyte	14	Atretic corpus luteum
11	Ruptured follicle	15	Corpus albicans
12	Atretic follicle		

FIGURE 5-8   Blood Supply of the Female Canine Reproductive Tract

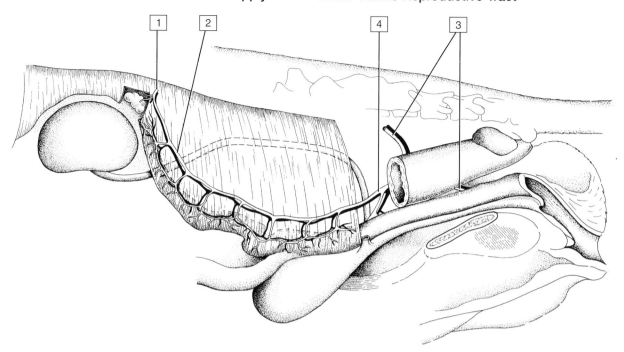

| 1 | Ovarian a. | 3 | Vaginal a. |
| 2 | Uterine branch of the ovarian a. | 4 | Uterine a. |

FIGURE 5-9   Formation of Canine Extraembryonic Membranes

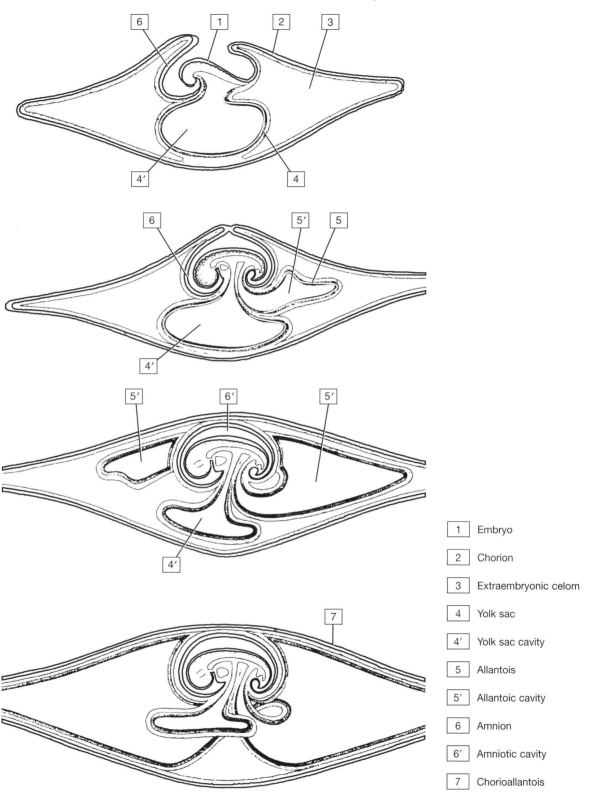

1	Embryo
2	Chorion
3	Extraembryonic celom
4	Yolk sac
4′	Yolk sac cavity
5	Allantois
5′	Allantoic cavity
6	Amnion
6′	Amniotic cavity
7	Chorioallantois

FIGURE 5-10   Transverse Section of the
Canine Pelvis at the Level of the Hip Joint

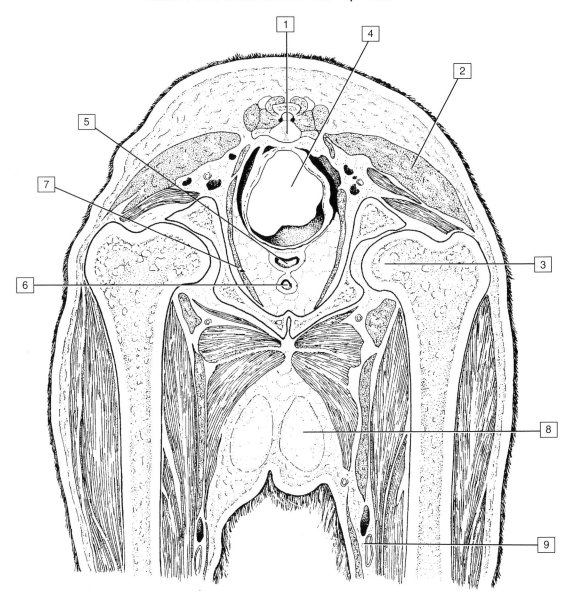

1	Caudal vertebra	6	Urethra
2	Superficial gluteal muscle	7	Levator ani
3	Head of femur in acetabulum	8	Inguinal mammary gland
4	Rectum suspended by a short mesorectum	9	Femoral a. and v.
5	Vagina		

FIGURE 5-11   Deep Dissection of the External Canine Reproductive Organs

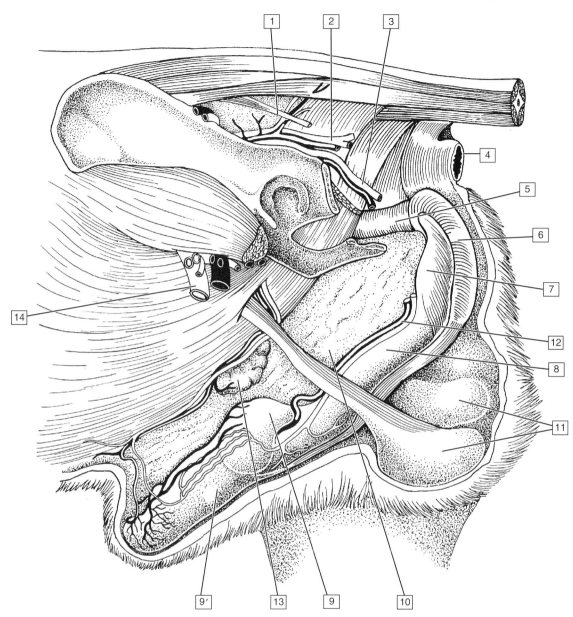

1	Sacrotuberous ligament	9	Bulbus glandis
2	Caudal gluteal vessels	9′	Pars longa glandis
3	Internal pudendal vessels	10	Spermatic cord
4	Anus	11	Testes in scrotum
5	Pelvic urethra	12	Dorsal artery and vein of the penis
6	Bulb of penis enclosed by Bulbospongiosus	13	Superficial inguinal lymph nodes and caudal superficial epigastric vessels
7	Ischiocavernosus over left crus	14	Femoral vessels
8	Body of penis		

FIGURE 5-12 Right Canine Lumbosacral Nerves and Left Arteries, Ventral View

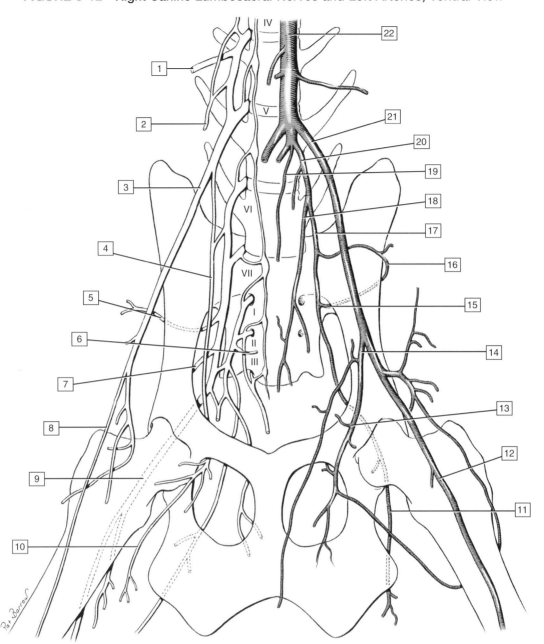

1	Lateral cutaneous femoral nerve	7	Caudal gluteal nerve	13	Medial circumflex femoral artery	18	Internal pudendal artery
2	Genitofemoral nerve	8	Saphenous nerve	14	Deep femoral artery	19	Median sacral artery
3	Femoral nerve	9	Sciatic nerve	15	Cranial gluteal artery	20	Internal iliac artery
4	Obturator nerve	10	Obturator nerve	16	Iliolumbar artery	21	External iliac artery
5	Cranial gluteal nerve	11	Caudal gluteal nerve	17	Caudal gluteal artery	22	Aorta
6	Pelvic nerve	12	Femoral artery				

FIGURE 5-13 Canine Nerves, Arteries, and
Muscles of the Right Hip, Lateral Aspect

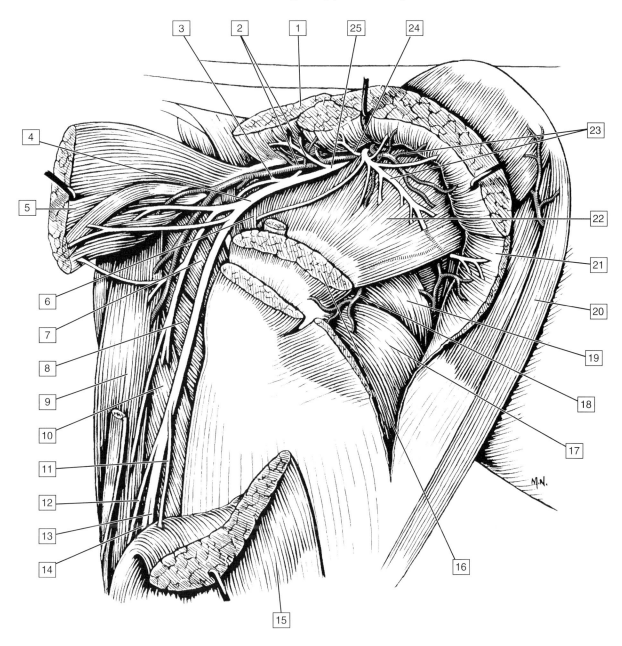

1	Superficial gluteus	7	Quadratus femoris	13	Common fibular nerve	20 Sartorius
2	Caudal gluteal artery and nerve	8	Adductor	14	Tibial nerve	21 Tensor fasciae latae
3	Nerve to internal obturator, gemelli, and quadratus femoris	9	Semitendinosus	15	Biceps femoris	22 Deep gluteal
		10	Semimembranosus	16	Middle gluteal	23 Cranial gluteal artery and nerve
4	Sciatic nerve	11	Lateral cutaneous sural nerve	17	Vastus lateralis	24 Nerve to piriformis
5	Biceps femoris	12	Caudal cutaneous sural nerve	18	Lateral circumflex femoral artery	25 Lumbosacral trunk
6	Gemelli			19	Rectus femoris	

FIGURE 5-14   The Reproductive Organs of the Tomcat in situ, Left Lateral View

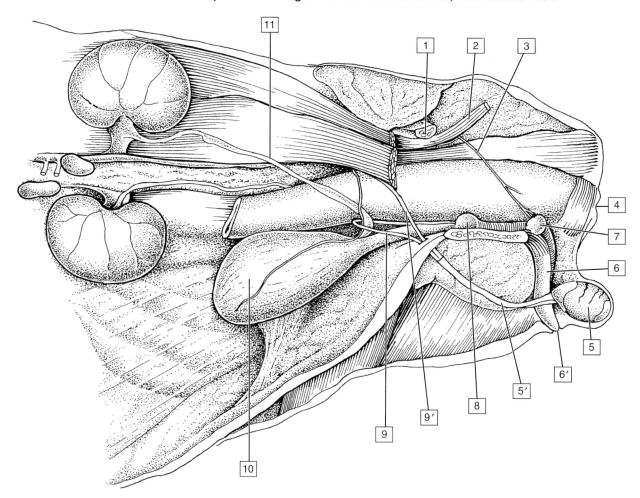

1	Shaft of ilium	6′	Prepuce
2	Sciatic nerve	7	Bulbourethral gland
3	Pudendal nerve	8	Prostate
4	Anus	9	Deferent duct
5	Left testis in scrotum	9′	Testicular vessels
5′	Spermatic cord	10	Bladder
6	Penis	11	Left ureter

FIGURE 5-15   Median Section of the Pelvis of the Mare and
Caudal Abdominal and Pelvic Organs of the Mare in situ

The organs have been sectioned in a paramedian plane with the
pelvis. Because of the absence of the intestines, the ovaries
hang much lower than they would in the intact animal.

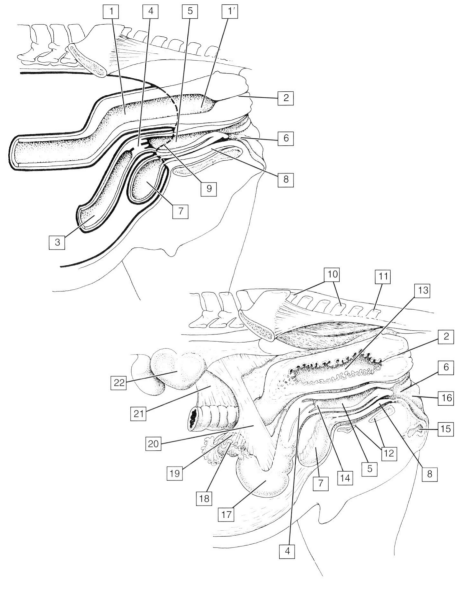

1 Peritoneal part of the rectum	6 Vestibule	12 Floor of pelvis	18 Uterine tube
1′ Retroperitoneal parts of the rectum	7 Bladder	13 Rectum	19 Ovary
2 Anal canal	8 Urethra	14 Vaginal part of cervix	20 Broad ligament (largely cut away)
3 Uterus	9 Caudal extent of peritoneum	15 Clitoris	21 Descending mesocolon
4 Cervix	10 Sacrum	16 Vulva	22 Left kidney
5 Vagina	11 Cd2	17 Left uterine horn	

FIGURE 5-16   Sacrum and Caudal Lumbar Vertebrae with
Emerging Ventral Rami Forming the Lumbosacral Plexus, Ventral View

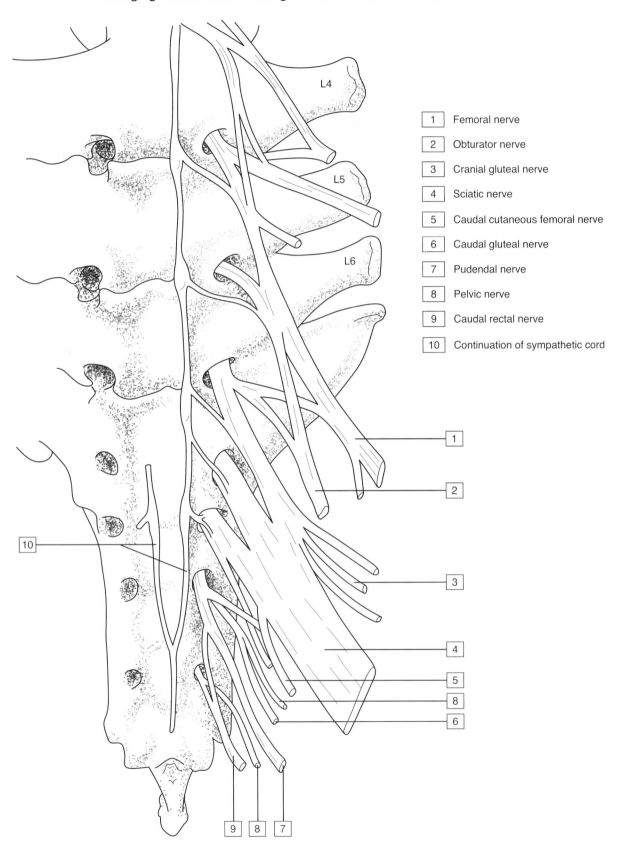

1	Femoral nerve
2	Obturator nerve
3	Cranial gluteal nerve
4	Sciatic nerve
5	Caudal cutaneous femoral nerve
6	Caudal gluteal nerve
7	Pudendal nerve
8	Pelvic nerve
9	Caudal rectal nerve
10	Continuation of sympathetic cord

Saunders Veterinary Anatomy Coloring Book

FIGURE 5-17

Equine right ovary, uterine tube, and uterine horn, lateral view

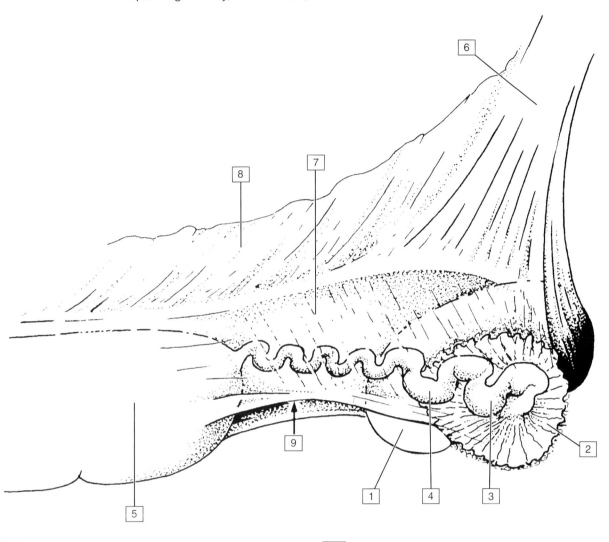

1	Ovary		6	Mesovarium
2	Infundibulum with fimbriae		7	Mesosalpinx
3	Ampulla of uterine tube		8	Mesometrium
4	Isthmus of uterine tube		9	Entrance to the ovarian bursa
5	Uterine horn			

FIGURE 5-18

Branching pattern of the caudal part of
the bovine abdominal aorta and the regional nodes

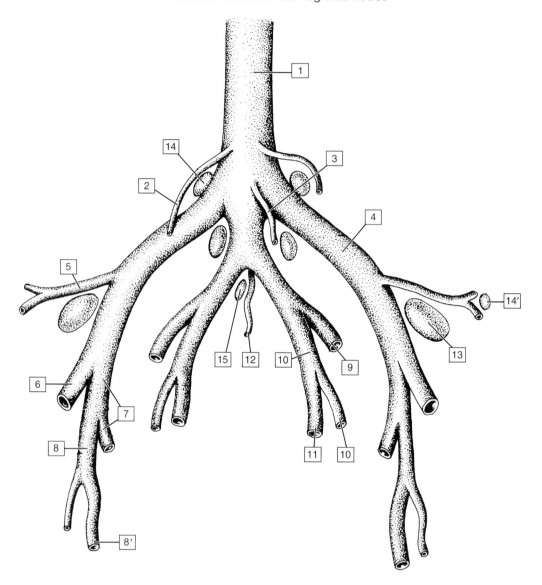

1	Aorta	9	Internal iliac artery
2	Ovarian a.	10	Umbilical artery
3	Caudal mesenteric a.	11	Uterine artery
4	External iliac a.	12	Median sacral artery
5	Deep circumflex iliac a.	13	Deep inguinal (iliofemoral) lymph node
6	Femoral a.	14	Medial iliac lymph node
7	Deep femoral a.	14'	Lateral iliac lymph nodes
8	Pudendoepigastric trunk	15	Sacral lymph nodes
8'	External pudendal artery		

FIGURE 5-19

Paramedian section of the caudal
abdomen and pelvis of a pregnant cow

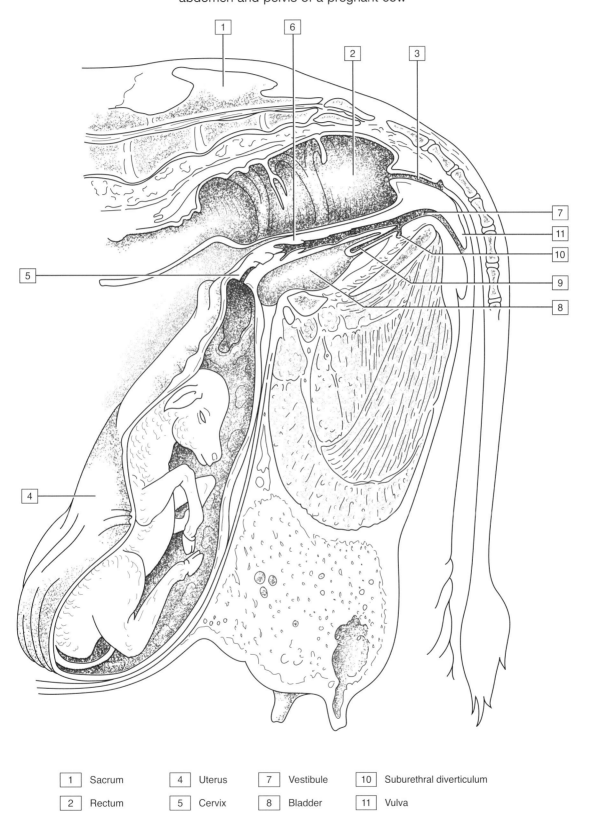

1	Sacrum	4	Uterus	7	Vestibule	10	Suburethral diverticulum
2	Rectum	5	Cervix	8	Bladder	11	Vulva
3	Anal canal	6	Vagina	9	Urethra		

FIGURE 5-20

Nerves and vessels on the
medial surface of the bovine pelvic wall

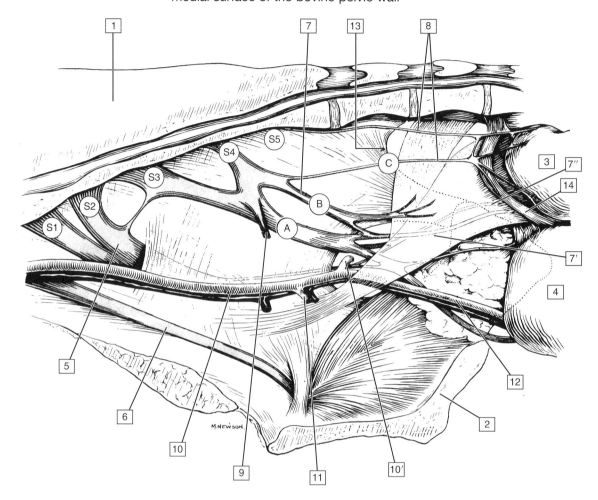

Local anesthesia of the pudendal nerve can be obtained
by injections at A and B. Anesthesia of the caudal rectal
nerves is possible by injection at C.

1 Sacrum	8 Caudal rectal n.
2 Pelvic symphysis	9 Pelvic n.
3 Rectum (reflected)	10 Internal iliac a.
4 Vagina (reflected)	10′ Caudal gluteal a.
5 Sciatic n.	11 Vaginal a.
6 Obturator n.	12 Internal pudendal a.
7 Pudendal n.	13 Caudal border of sacrosciatic ligament
7′ Distal cutaneous branch of pudendal n.	14 Retractor clitoridis
7″ Proximal cutaneous branch of pudendal n.	

FIGURE 5-21 The Bovine Reproductive Organs, Dorsal View

The uterus, cervix, vagina, and vestibule have been opened.

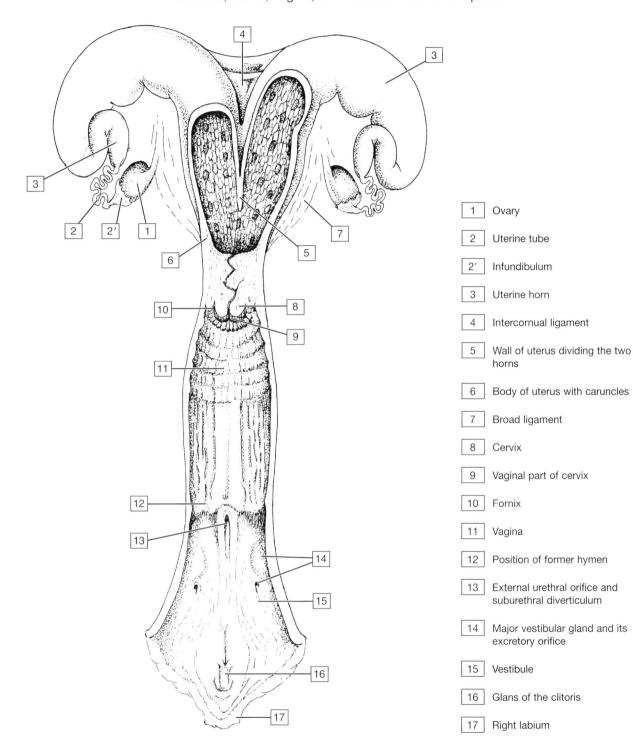

1	Ovary
2	Uterine tube
2'	Infundibulum
3	Uterine horn
4	Intercornual ligament
5	Wall of uterus dividing the two horns
6	Body of uterus with caruncles
7	Broad ligament
8	Cervix
9	Vaginal part of cervix
10	Fornix
11	Vagina
12	Position of former hymen
13	External urethral orifice and suburethral diverticulum
14	Major vestibular gland and its excretory orifice
15	Vestibule
16	Glans of the clitoris
17	Right labium

FIGURE 5-22

Semischematic of the blood
supply to bovine reproductive tract, ventral view

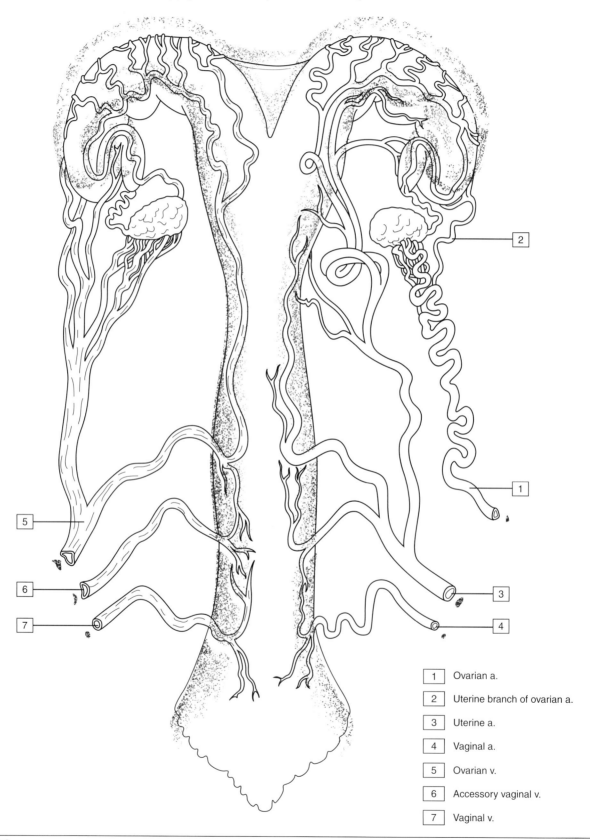

1	Ovarian a.
2	Uterine branch of ovarian a.
3	Uterine a.
4	Vaginal a.
5	Ovarian v.
6	Accessory vaginal v.
7	Vaginal v.

Saunders Veterinary Anatomy Coloring Book

FIGURE 5-23

The bovine penis and its muscles; caudolateral view

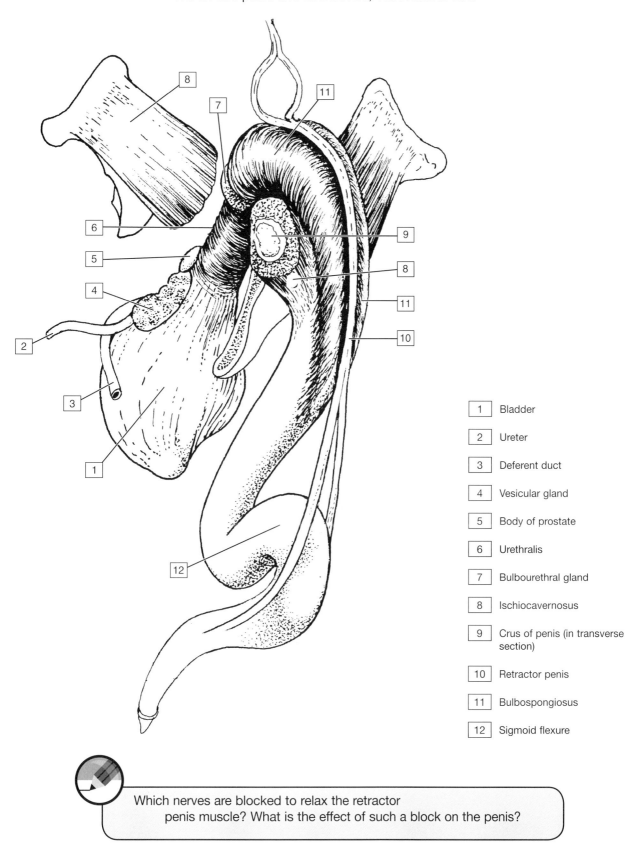

1	Bladder
2	Ureter
3	Deferent duct
4	Vesicular gland
5	Body of prostate
6	Urethralis
7	Bulbourethral gland
8	Ischiocavernosus
9	Crus of penis (in transverse section)
10	Retractor penis
11	Bulbospongiosus
12	Sigmoid flexure

Which nerves are blocked to relax the retractor penis muscle? What is the effect of such a block on the penis?

FIGURE 5-24   Developing Duct Systems
Growing Proximally from the Tip of the Fetal Teat

A, Cow, ewe, and goat. *B,* Mare and sow.
C, Bitch and cat (only four primary sprouts are shown).

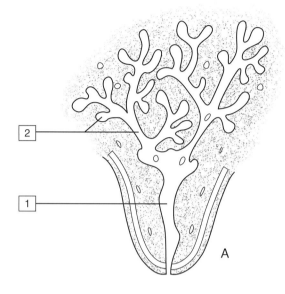

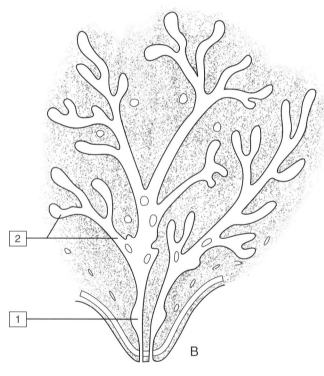

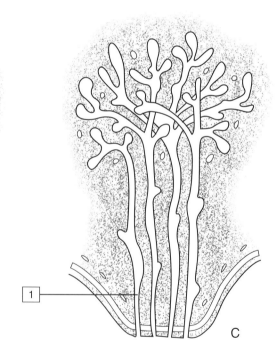

1   Primary sprout   2   Secondary and tertiary sprouts

Saunders Veterinary Anatomy Coloring Book

FIGURE 5-25

Bovine venous and lymph drainage of the udder

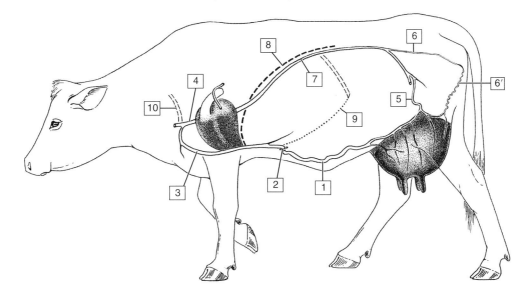

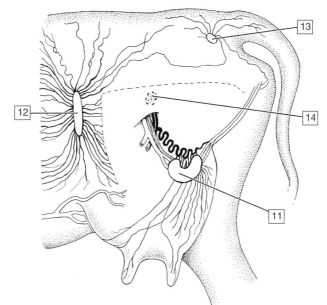

1	Subcutaneous abdominal (milk) v.		8	Diaphragm
2	Milk "well"		9	Costal arch
3	Internal thoracic v.		10	First rib
4	Cranial vena cava		11	Mammary (superficial inguinal) lymph node
5	External pudendal v.		12	Subiliac lymph node
6	Internal pudendal v.		13	Ischial lymph node
6'	Ventral labial v. (connecting ventral perineal v. with caudal mammary veins)		14	Position of deep inguinal (iliofemoral) node
7	Caudal vena cava			

FIGURE 5-26   Cranial View of the Opened Scrotum of a Bull

The investments of the testis have been partly dissected.

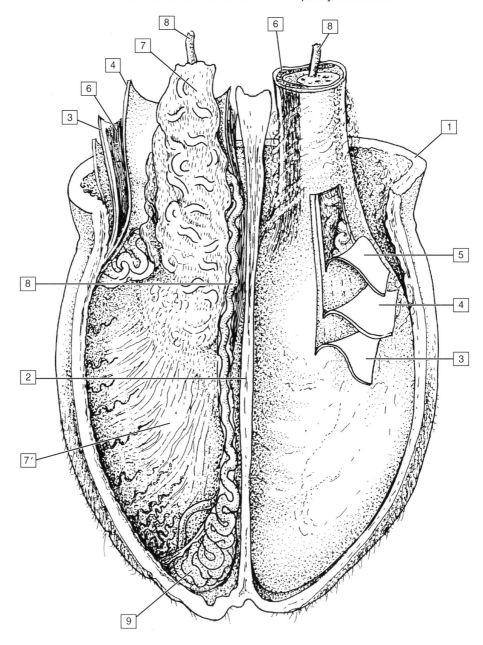

1	Scrotal skin and dartos
2	Scrotal septum
3	External spermatic fascia
4	Parietal layer of vaginal tunic
5	Visceral layer (dissected from surface of testis)
6	Cremaster muscle

7	Visceral layer of vaginal tunic covering structures in spermatic cord
7'	Visceral layer on testis
8	Deferent duct
9	Tail of epididymis

The pronephric duct drains the mesonephros
and is now more aptly termed the *mesonephric duct*.

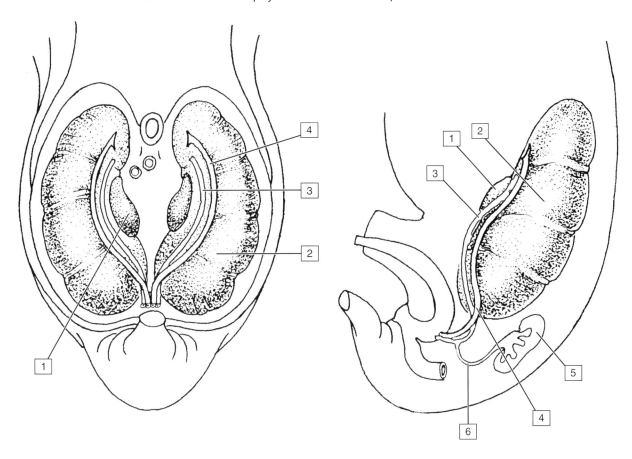

1	Developing gonad	4	Paramesonephric duct
2	Mesonephros	5	Metanephros
3	Mesonephric duct	6	Ureter

FIGURE 5-28   The Development of the Metanephros
from Two Primordia (Metanephric Cord and Ureteric Bud)

Note the gradual regression of the mesonephros.

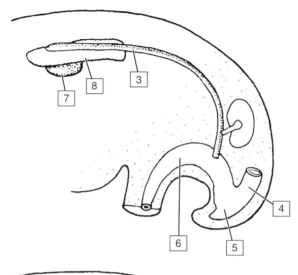
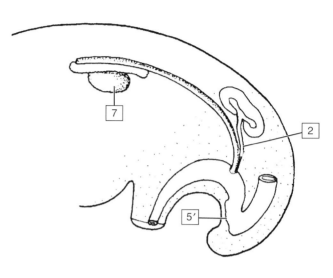
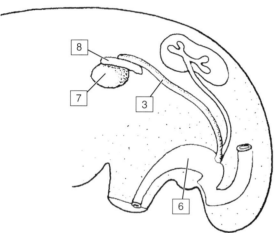
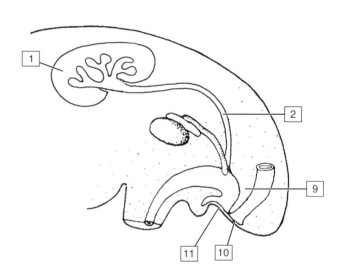

1	Metanephros	6	Urogenital sinus
2	Ureteric bud (future ureter)	7	Gonad
3	Mesonephric (deferent) duct	8	Remnant of mesonephros (future epididymis)
4	Rectum	9	Urorectal septum
5	Cloaca	10	Anal membrane
5′	Cloacal membrane	11	Urogenital membrane

FIGURE 5-29   Transverse Section of the Free End of the Porcine Penis

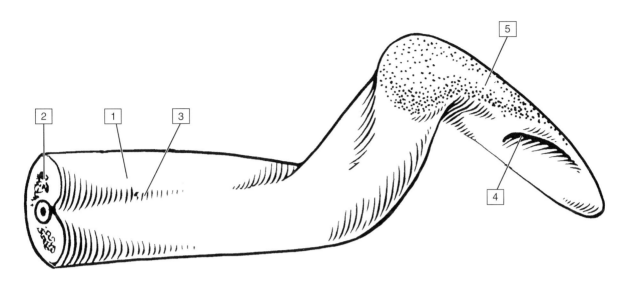

1	Tunica albuginea		4	External urethral orifice
2	Corpus cavernosum		5	Thin glans penis
3	Urethral groove			

6 THE FORELIMB

FIGURE 6-1

Canine left humerus, cranial view

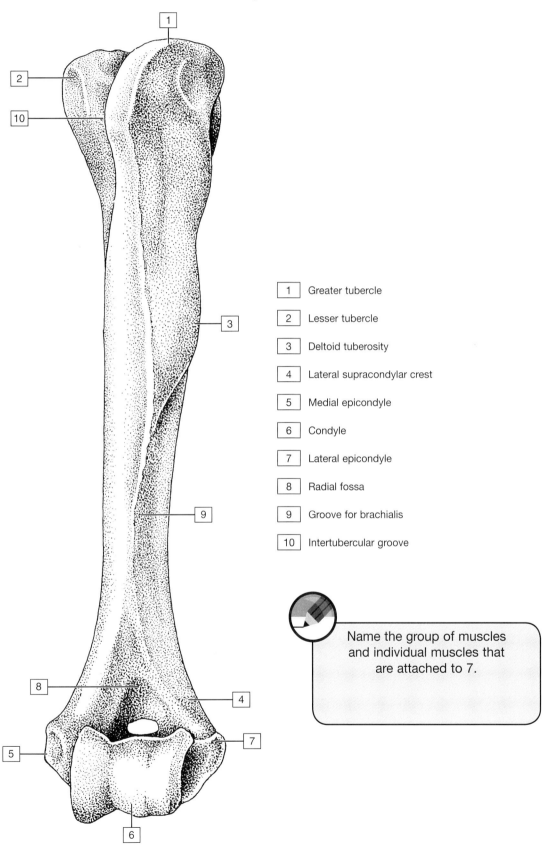

1	Greater tubercle
2	Lesser tubercle
3	Deltoid tuberosity
4	Lateral supracondylar crest
5	Medial epicondyle
6	Condyle
7	Lateral epicondyle
8	Radial fossa
9	Groove for brachialis
10	Intertubercular groove

Name the group of muscles and individual muscles that are attached to 7.

FIGURE 6-2

Canine left ulna and left radius

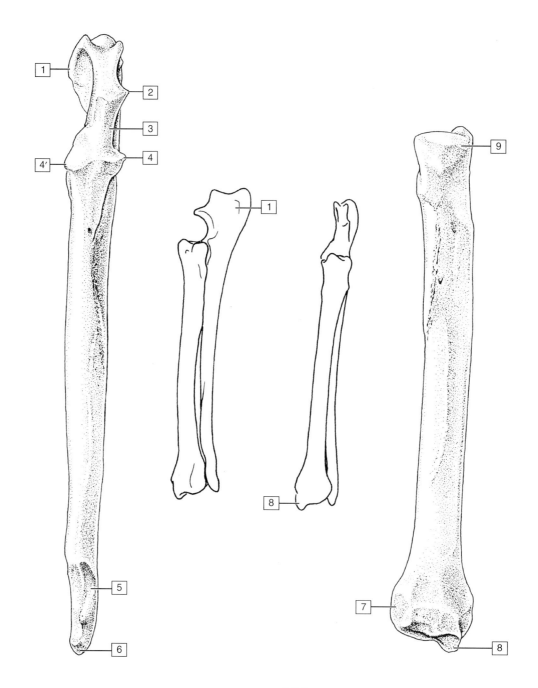

1	Olecranon
2	Anconeal process
3	Trochlear notch
4	Lateral coronoid process
4'	Medial coronoid process
5	Distal articular facet for radius

6	Lateral styloid process (with facet for the ulnar carpal bone in the dog)
7	Articular facet for ulna
8	Medial styloid process
9	Circumferential facet

FIGURE 6-3

Superficial muscles of the canine shoulder and arm

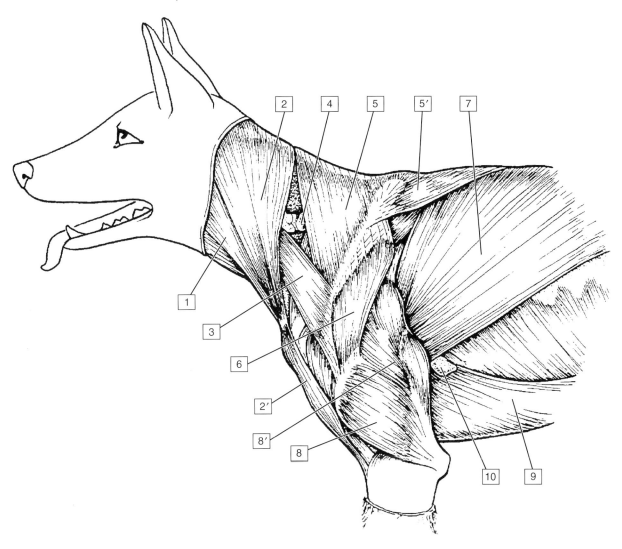

1	Sternocephalicus	6	Deltoideus
2	Brachiocephalicus: cleidocervicalis	7	Latissimus dorsi
2′	Brachiocephalicus: cleidobrachialis	8	Lateral head of triceps
3	Omotransversarius	8′	Long head of triceps
4	Superficial cervical lymph node	9	Pectoralis profundus (ascendens)
5	Cervical part of trapezius	10	Accessory axillary lymph node
5′	Thoracic part of trapezius		

Name the group or muscles that attaches to number 7.

FIGURE 6-4

Intrinsic muscles of the canine left shoulder and arm, lateral and medial views

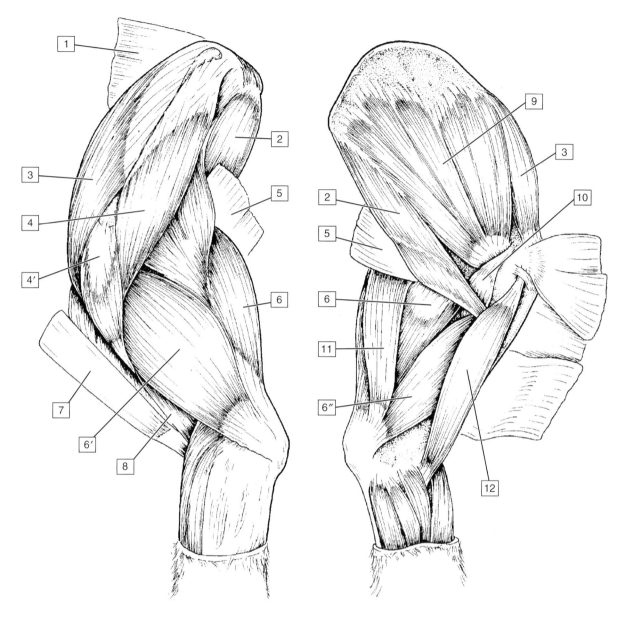

1	Rhomboideus	6''	Medial head of triceps
2	Teres major	7	Brachiocephalicus
3	Supraspinatus	8	Brachialis
4	Scapular part of deltoideus	9	Subscapularis
4'	Acromial part of deltoideus	10	Coracobrachialis
5	Latissimus dorsi	11	Tensor fasciae antebrachii
6	Long head of triceps	12	Biceps
6'	Lateral head of triceps		

FIGURE 6-5 Axial Section of the Paw

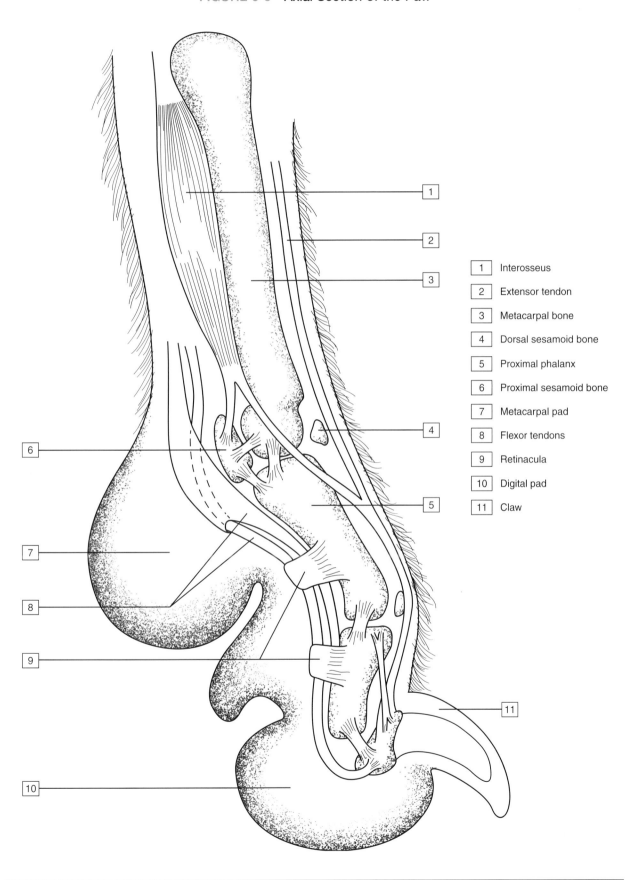

1	Interosseus
2	Extensor tendon
3	Metacarpal bone
4	Dorsal sesamoid bone
5	Proximal phalanx
6	Proximal sesamoid bone
7	Metacarpal pad
8	Flexor tendons
9	Retinacula
10	Digital pad
11	Claw

FIGURE 6-6

Muscles of the canine left forearm, lateral and medial views

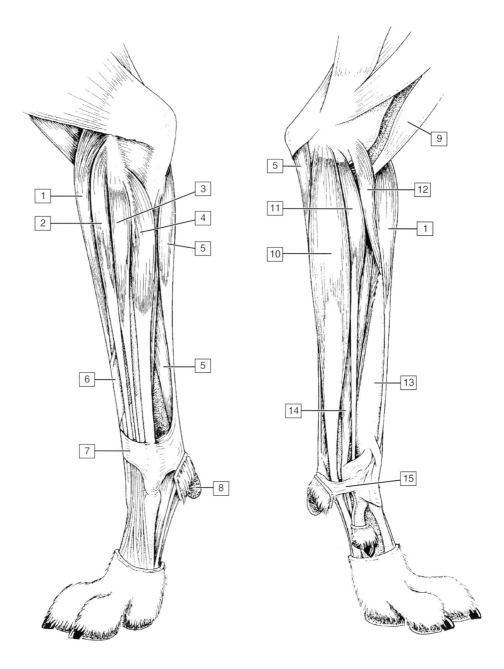

1 Extensor carpi radialis	6 Extensor carpi obliquus	11 Flexor carpi radialis
2 Common digital extensor	7 Extensor retinaculum	12 Pronator teres
3 Lateral digital extensor	8 Carpal pad	13 Radius
4 Ulnaris lateralis	9 Biceps	14 Deep digital flexor
5 Flexor carpi ulnaris	10 Superficial digital flexor	15 Flexor retinaculum

FIGURE 6-7   Transverse Section of the Left
Canine Forelimb Just Distal to the Shoulder Joint

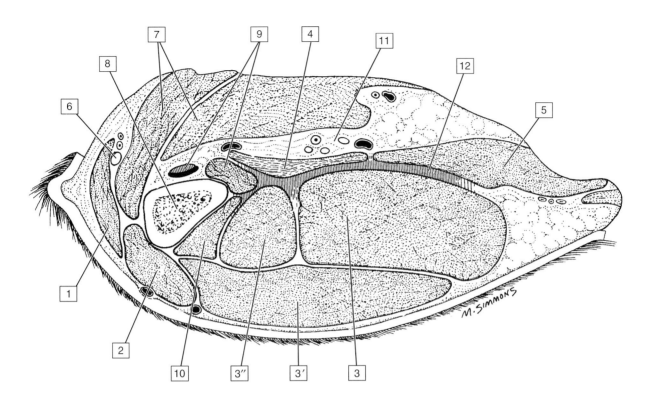

1	Brachiocephalicus	
2	Deltoideus	
3	Long head of triceps	
3'	Lateral head of triceps	
3''	Accessory head of triceps	
4	Teres major	
5	Latissimus dorsi	

6	Cephalic vein
7	Pectoral muscles
8	Humerus
9	Biceps tendon and coracobrachialis
10	Brachialis
11	Brachial vessels and nerve trunks
12	Heavy intermuscular fascia

FIGURE 6-8

Superficial veins on the left canine forearm

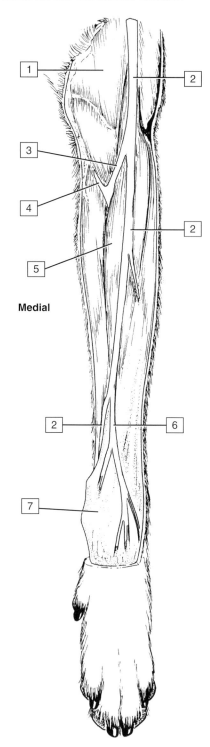

Medial

1	Brachiocephalicus	
2	Cephalic v.	
3	Median cubital v.	
4	Brachial v.	
5	Extensor carpi radialis	
6	Accessory cephalic v.	
7	Carpus	

Saunders Veterinary Anatomy Coloring Book

FIGURE 6-9

Transverse section of the left canine forelimb just proximal to the carpus

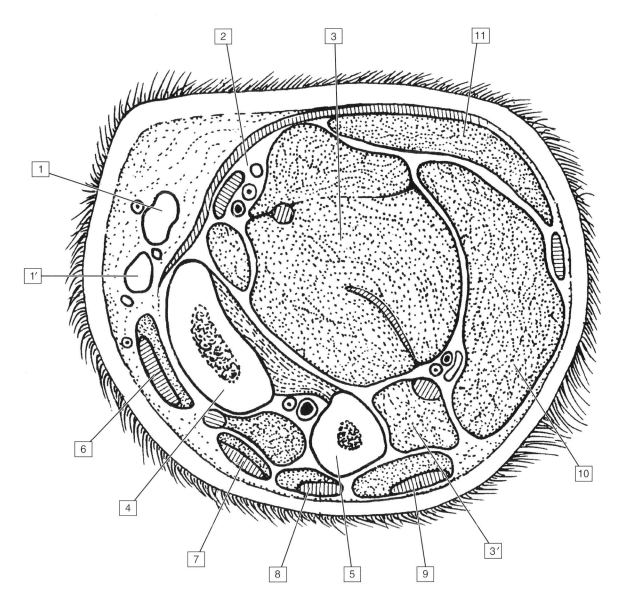

1	Cephalic vein and branches of superficial radial nerve
1′	Accessory cephalic vein
2	Median vessels and nerve and flexor carpi radialis
3	Humeral head of deep digital flexor
3′	Ulnar head of deep digital flexor
4	Radius
5	Ulna

6	Extensor carpi radialis
7	Common digital extensor
8	Lateral digital extensor
9	Ulnaris lateralis
10	Flexor carpi ulnaris: its small ulnar head lies on its caudal aspects, and the ulnar vessels and nerve on its cranial aspect
11	Superficial digital flexor

FIGURE 6-10 Topography of the Major Arteries
of the Right Canine Forelimb, Medial View

The caudomedial muscles of the forearm have been removed.

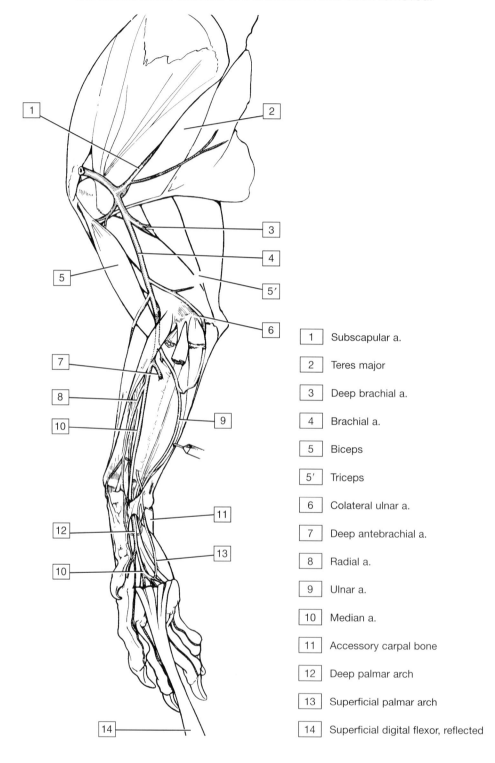

1	Subscapular a.
2	Teres major
3	Deep brachial a.
4	Brachial a.
5	Biceps
5′	Triceps
6	Colateral ulnar a.
7	Deep antebrachial a.
8	Radial a.
9	Ulnar a.
10	Median a.
11	Accessory carpal bone
12	Deep palmar arch
13	Superficial palmar arch
14	Superficial digital flexor, reflected

FIGURE 6-11 The Blood Supply of a Canine Long Bone

The supply of the cortex is shown (enlarged) in the center.

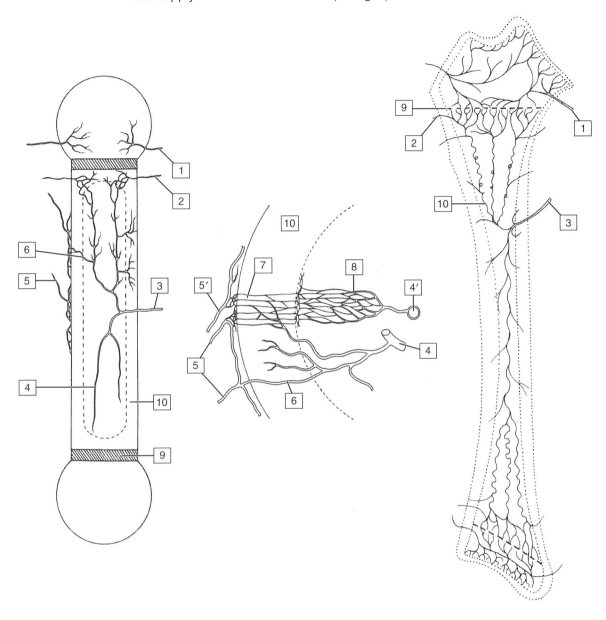

1	Epiphysial aa.	5'	Periosteal v.
2	Metaphysial aa.	6	Anastomosis between periosteal and bone marrow aa.
3	Nutrient a.	7	Capillaries of the cortex
4	Artery of the bone marrow	8	Sinusoids in the bone marrow
4'	Vein of the bone marrow	9	Growth cartilage
5	Periosteal aa.	10	Cortex

FIGURE 6-12   Cranial View of the Canine Left Stifle Joint

The joint is resected to show intracapsular and extracapsular ligaments.

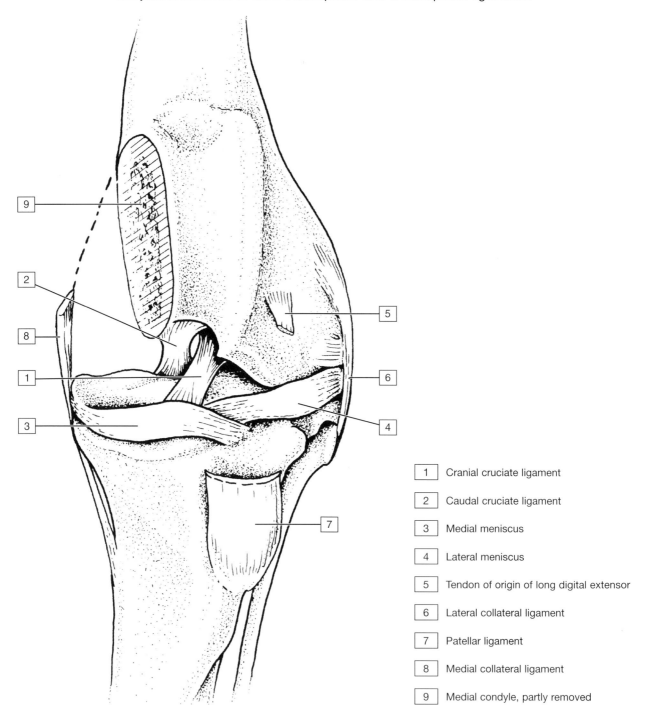

1	Cranial cruciate ligament
2	Caudal cruciate ligament
3	Medial meniscus
4	Lateral meniscus
5	Tendon of origin of long digital extensor
6	Lateral collateral ligament
7	Patellar ligament
8	Medial collateral ligament
9	Medial condyle, partly removed

FIGURE 6-13

Sections of a synovial bursa (*A*) and a tendon sheath
(*B*). The bursa permits frictionless movement of a tendon over
bone, the sheath movement of a tendon over bone and under a
retinaculum, respectively. The *arrows* show that a tendon sheath may
be regarded as a large bursa that has wrapped around a tendon.

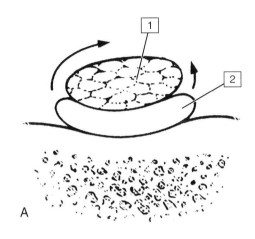

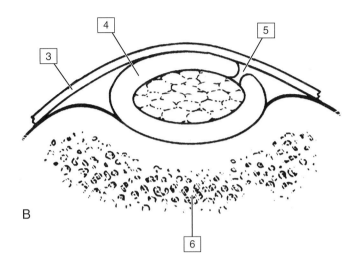

A

B

1	Tendon
2	Bursa
3	Retinaculum

4	Tendon sheath
5	Mesotendon, through which blood vessels reach the tendon
6	Bone

FIGURE 6-14

Canine left forelimb skeleton, lateral view of muscle attachments

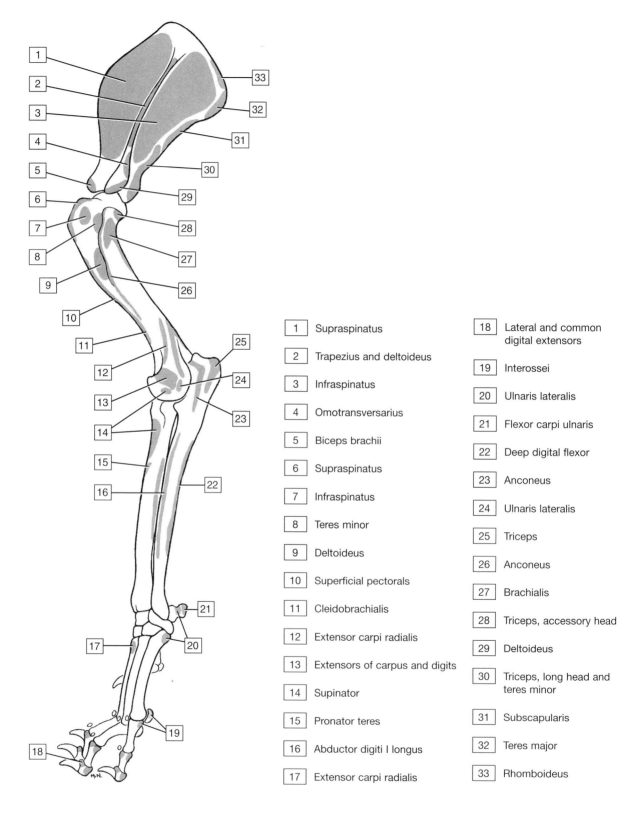

1	Supraspinatus	18	Lateral and common digital extensors
2	Trapezius and deltoideus	19	Interossei
3	Infraspinatus	20	Ulnaris lateralis
4	Omotransversarius	21	Flexor carpi ulnaris
5	Biceps brachii	22	Deep digital flexor
6	Supraspinatus	23	Anconeus
7	Infraspinatus	24	Ulnaris lateralis
8	Teres minor	25	Triceps
9	Deltoideus	26	Anconeus
10	Superficial pectorals	27	Brachialis
11	Cleidobrachialis	28	Triceps, accessory head
12	Extensor carpi radialis	29	Deltoideus
13	Extensors of carpus and digits	30	Triceps, long head and teres minor
14	Supinator	31	Subscapularis
15	Pronator teres	32	Teres major
16	Abductor digiti I longus	33	Rhomboideus
17	Extensor carpi radialis		

FIGURE 6-15   Major Extensors and Flexors of the Canine Left Forelimb

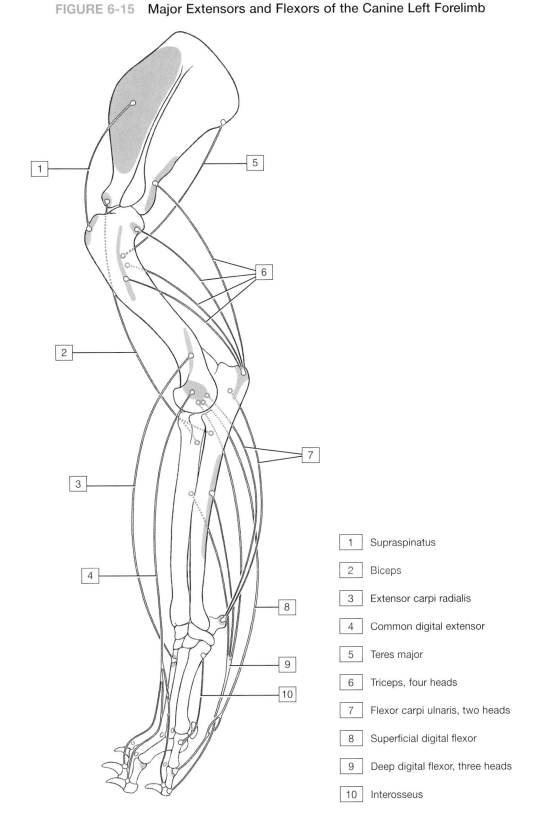

1	Supraspinatus
2	Biceps
3	Extensor carpi radialis
4	Common digital extensor
5	Teres major
6	Triceps, four heads
7	Flexor carpi ulnaris, two heads
8	Superficial digital flexor
9	Deep digital flexor, three heads
10	Interosseus

FIGURE 6-16

A, Distribution of canine musculocutaneous and median nerves, right forelimb, medial view. *B,* Distribution of canine radial nerve, right forelimb, lateral view.

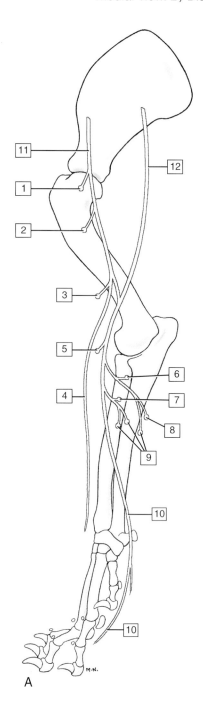

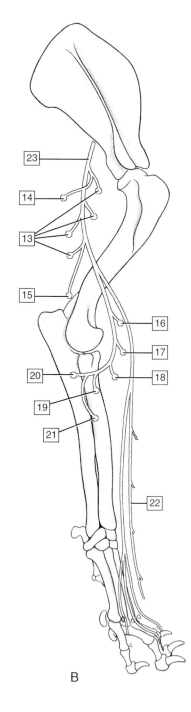

Musculocutaneous nerve

1   Coracobrachialis

2   Biceps brachii

3   Brachialis

4   Skin of medial antebrachium

Median nerve

5   Pronator teres

6   Flexor carpi radialis

7   Pronator quadratus

8   Superficial digital flexor

9   Deep digital flexor, humeral, ulnar and radial heads

10   Skin of caudal antebrachium and palmar paw

11   Musculocutaneous nerve

12   Median nerve

Radial nerve

13   Triceps brachii

14   Tensor fasciae antebrachii

15   Anconeus

16   Extensor carpi radialis

17   Supinator

18   Common digital extensor

19   Lateral digital extensor

20   Ulnaris lateralis

21   Abductor digiti I longus

22   Skin of cranial and lateral antebrachium and dorsal paw

23   Radial nerve

A

B

FIGURE 6-17

Distribution of canine ulnar nerve, right forelimb, medial view

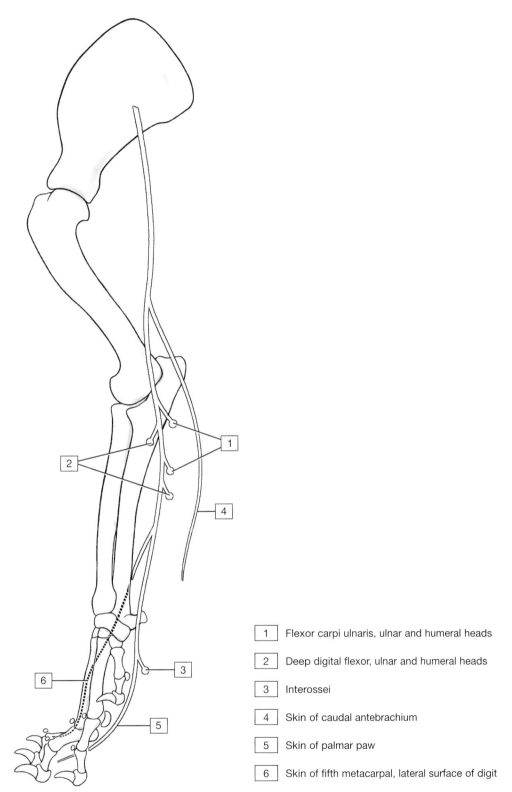

1	Flexor carpi ulnaris, ulnar and humeral heads
2	Deep digital flexor, ulnar and humeral heads
3	Interossei
4	Skin of caudal antebrachium
5	Skin of palmar paw
6	Skin of fifth metacarpal, lateral surface of digit

FIGURE 6-18

Veins of canine right forelimb, schematic medial view

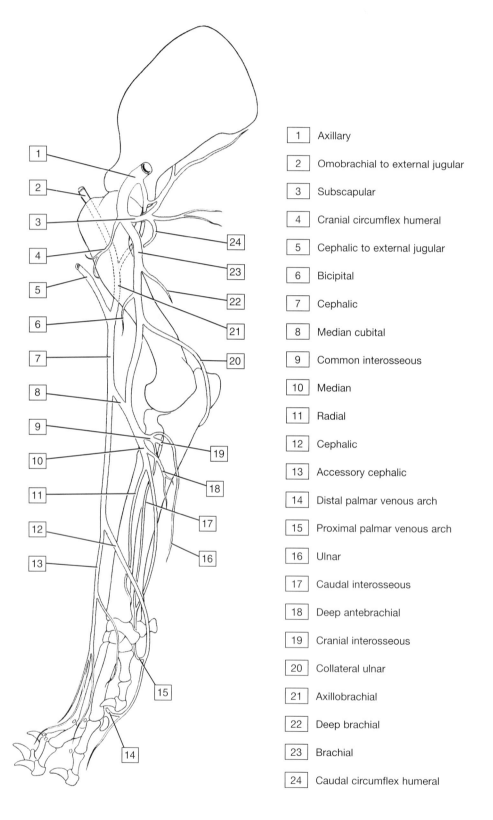

1	Axillary
2	Omobrachial to external jugular
3	Subscapular
4	Cranial circumflex humeral
5	Cephalic to external jugular
6	Bicipital
7	Cephalic
8	Median cubital
9	Common interosseous
10	Median
11	Radial
12	Cephalic
13	Accessory cephalic
14	Distal palmar venous arch
15	Proximal palmar venous arch
16	Ulnar
17	Caudal interosseous
18	Deep antebrachial
19	Cranial interosseous
20	Collateral ulnar
21	Axillobrachial
22	Deep brachial
23	Brachial
24	Caudal circumflex humeral

FIGURE 6-19   Equine Superficial Muscles and Veins

The cutaneous muscles except for the cutaneous colli have been removed.

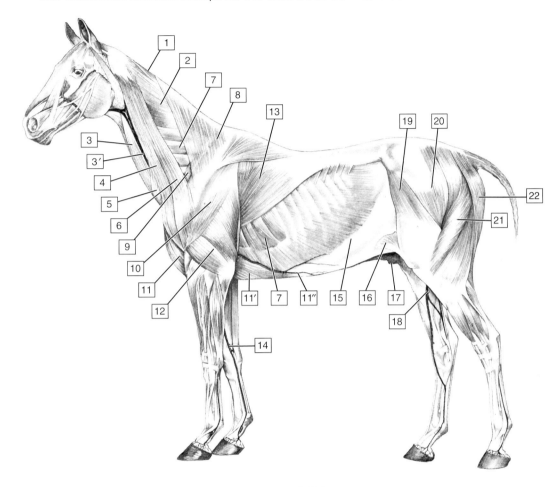

1 Rhomboideus	11″ Superficial thoracic vein
2 Splenius	12 Triceps
3 Sternocephalicus	13 Latissimus dorsi
3′ Jugular vein	14 Cephalic vein
4 Brachiocephalicus	15 External abdominal oblique
5 Cutaneous colli	16 Stump of cutaneus trunci forming flank fold
6 Omotransversarius	17 Sheath
7 Serratus ventralis	18 Medial saphenous vein
8 Trapezius	19 Tensor fasciae latae
9 Subclavius	20 Gluteus superficialis
10 Deltoideus	21 Biceps femoris
11 Pectoralis descendens	22 Semitendinosus
11′ Pectoralis ascendens	

FIGURE 6-20

Muscles on the ventral surface of the equine thorax

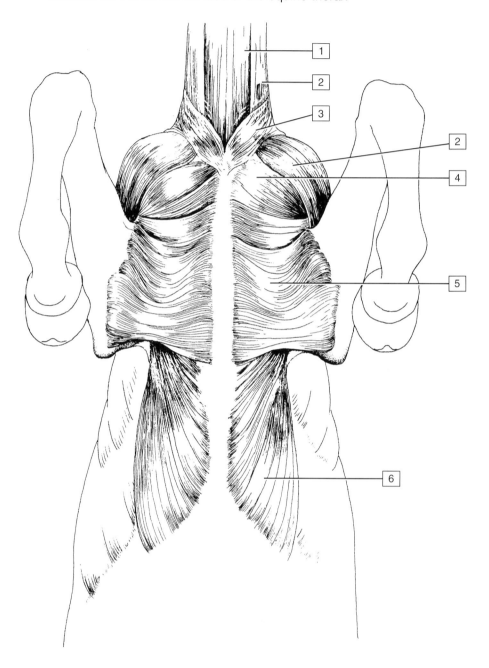

1	Sternocephalicus
2	Brachiocephalicus
3	Cutaneous colli

4	Pectoralis descendens
5	Pectoralis transversus
6	Pectoralis profundus

FIGURE 6-21

Deep muscles attaching the equine forelimb to the trunk

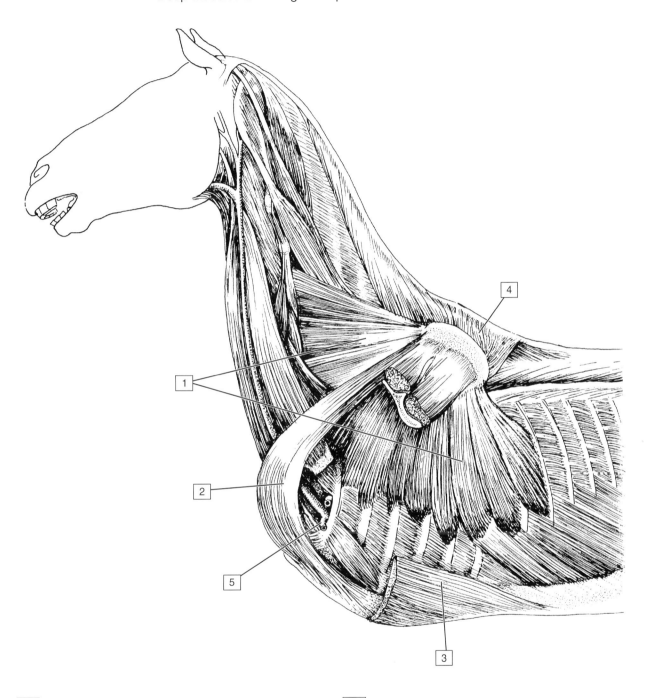

1	Serratus ventralis	4	Rhomboideus
2	Subclavius	5	Axillary vessels turning around first rib into limb
3	Pectoralis profundus		

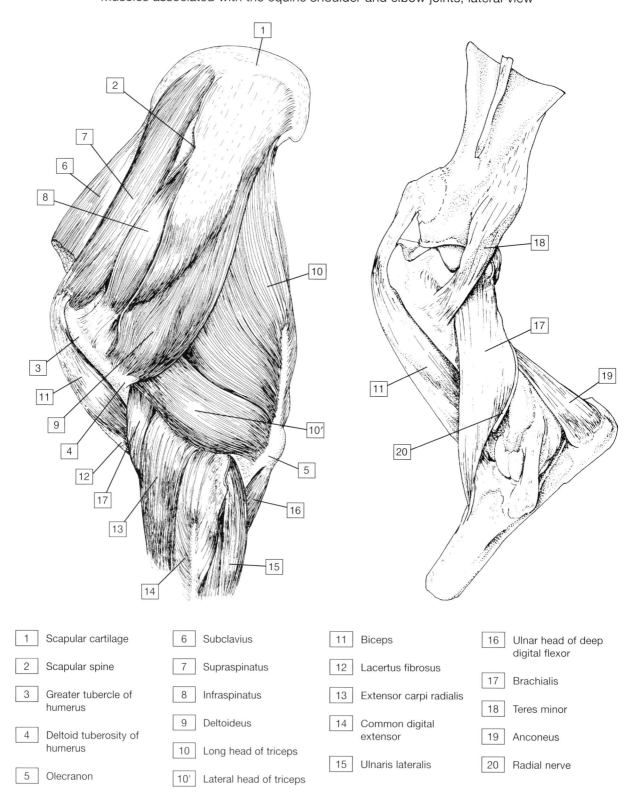

FIGURE 6-22

Muscles associated with the equine shoulder and elbow joints; lateral view

1	Scapular cartilage	6	Subclavius	11	Biceps	16	Ulnar head of deep digital flexor
2	Scapular spine	7	Supraspinatus	12	Lacertus fibrosus	17	Brachialis
3	Greater tubercle of humerus	8	Infraspinatus	13	Extensor carpi radialis	18	Teres minor
4	Deltoid tuberosity of humerus	9	Deltoideus	14	Common digital extensor	19	Anconeus
5	Olecranon	10	Long head of triceps	15	Ulnaris lateralis	20	Radial nerve
		10'	Lateral head of triceps				

Saunders Veterinary Anatomy Coloring Book

FIGURE 6-23

Nerve, arteries, and muscles on the medial surface of the equine right shoulder and arm

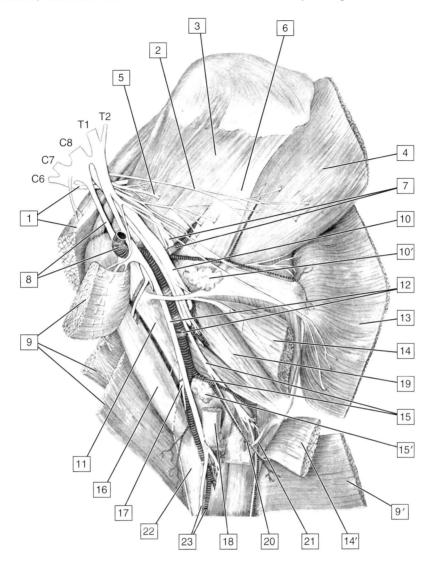

1	Suprascapular n. and subclavius	10	Radial n.	16	Biceps
2	Thoracodorsal n.	10'	Axillary lymph nodes	17	Musculocutaneous and medial cutaneous antebrachial nn.
3	Subscapularis	11	Coracobrachialis		
4	Latissimus dorsi	12	Median n. and brachial a.	18	Flexor carpi radialis
5	Subscapular n.	13	Cutaneous trunci	19	Triceps
6	Teres major	14	Stump of tensor fasciae antebrachii	20	Caudal cutaneous antebrachial n.
7	Axillary n. and subscapular a.	14'	Stump of tensor fasciae antebrachii	21	Flexor carpi ulnaris
8	Musculocutaneous n. and axillary a.			22	Lacertus fibrosus
9	Pectoralis profundus	15	Ulnar n. and collateral ulnar a.	23	Median n. and a.
9'	Pectoralis descendens	15'	Cubital lymph nodes		

FIGURE 6-24

Distal muscles of the equine left forelimb, medial view

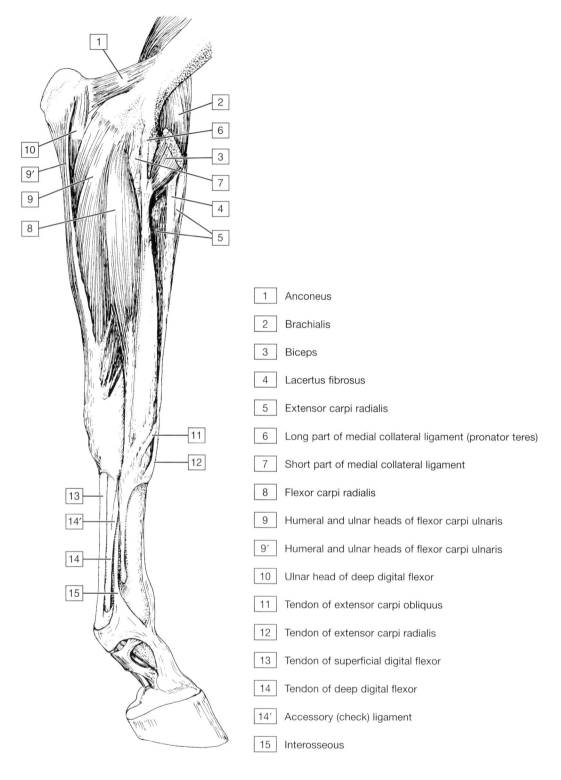

1	Anconeus
2	Brachialis
3	Biceps
4	Lacertus fibrosus
5	Extensor carpi radialis
6	Long part of medial collateral ligament (pronator teres)
7	Short part of medial collateral ligament
8	Flexor carpi radialis
9	Humeral and ulnar heads of flexor carpi ulnaris
9′	Humeral and ulnar heads of flexor carpi ulnaris
10	Ulnar head of deep digital flexor
11	Tendon of extensor carpi obliquus
12	Tendon of extensor carpi radialis
13	Tendon of superficial digital flexor
14	Tendon of deep digital flexor
14′	Accessory (check) ligament
15	Interosseous

FIGURE 6-25

Skeleton of the distal part of the equine left forelimb, dorsal view

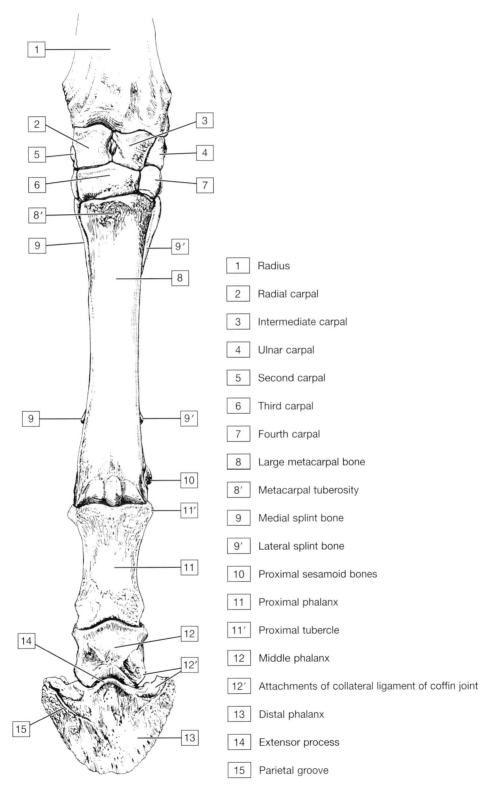

1	Radius
2	Radial carpal
3	Intermediate carpal
4	Ulnar carpal
5	Second carpal
6	Third carpal
7	Fourth carpal
8	Large metacarpal bone
8'	Metacarpal tuberosity
9	Medial splint bone
9'	Lateral splint bone
10	Proximal sesamoid bones
11	Proximal phalanx
11'	Proximal tubercle
12	Middle phalanx
12'	Attachments of collateral ligament of coffin joint
13	Distal phalanx
14	Extensor process
15	Parietal groove

FIGURE 6-26

Axial section of equine digit

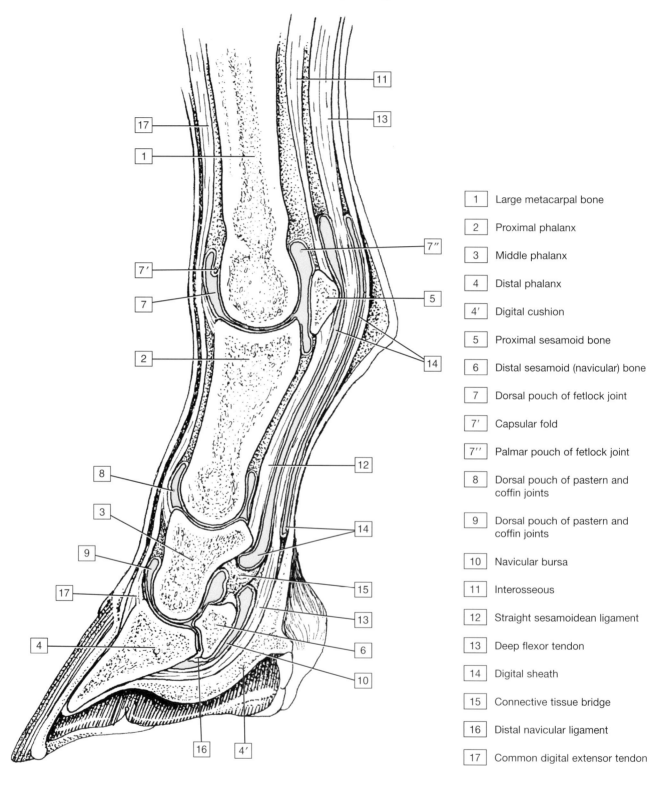

1	Large metacarpal bone
2	Proximal phalanx
3	Middle phalanx
4	Distal phalanx
4'	Digital cushion
5	Proximal sesamoid bone
6	Distal sesamoid (navicular) bone
7	Dorsal pouch of fetlock joint
7'	Capsular fold
7''	Palmar pouch of fetlock joint
8	Dorsal pouch of pastern and coffin joints
9	Dorsal pouch of pastern and coffin joints
10	Navicular bursa
11	Interosseous
12	Straight sesamoidean ligament
13	Deep flexor tendon
14	Digital sheath
15	Connective tissue bridge
16	Distal navicular ligament
17	Common digital extensor tendon

FIGURE 6-27

The major arteries of the equine right forelimb, palmar view

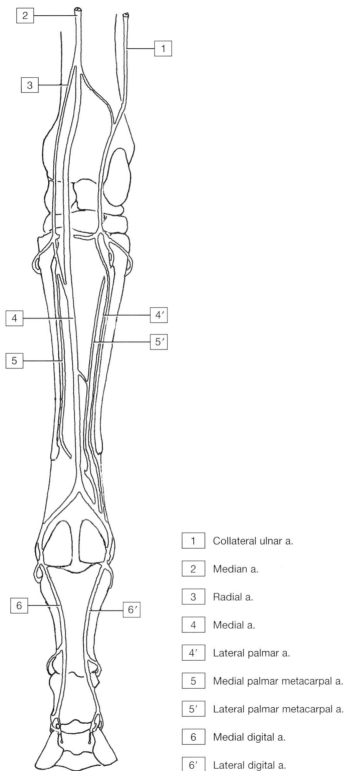

1	Collateral ulnar a.
2	Median a.
3	Radial a.
4	Medial a.
4'	Lateral palmar a.
5	Medial palmar metacarpal a.
5'	Lateral palmar metacarpal a.
6	Medial digital a.
6'	Lateral digital a.

FIGURE 6-28

Transverse section of the equine left elbow

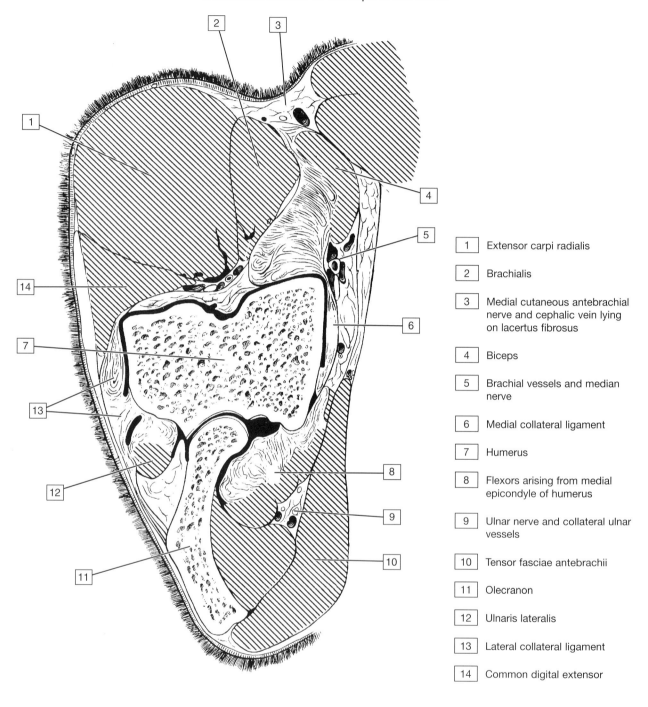

1 Extensor carpi radialis

2 Brachialis

3 Medial cutaneous antebrachial nerve and cephalic vein lying on lacertus fibrosus

4 Biceps

5 Brachial vessels and median nerve

6 Medial collateral ligament

7 Humerus

8 Flexors arising from medial epicondyle of humerus

9 Ulnar nerve and collateral ulnar vessels

10 Tensor fasciae antebrachii

11 Olecranon

12 Ulnaris lateralis

13 Lateral collateral ligament

14 Common digital extensor

Saunders Veterinary Anatomy Coloring Book

FIGURE 6-29

Transverse section of the middle of the bovine left forearm

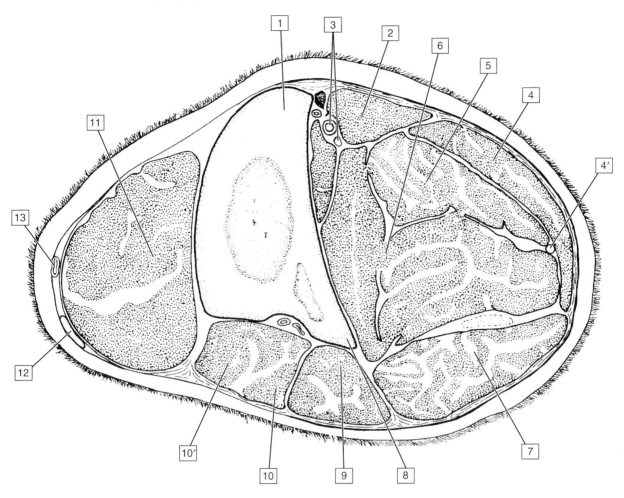

1	Radius	8	Ulna
2	Flexor carpi radialis	9	Lateral digital extensor
3	Median vessels and nerve	10	Common digital extensor
4	Flexor carpi ulnaris	10′	Common digital extensor
4′	Ulnar nerve	11	Extensor carpi radialis
5	Superficial digital flexor	12	Superficial branch of radial nerve
6	Deep digital flexor	13	Cephalic vein
7	Ulnaris lateralis		

FIGURE 6-30

Sagittal section of the bovine foot, splitting the lateral digit

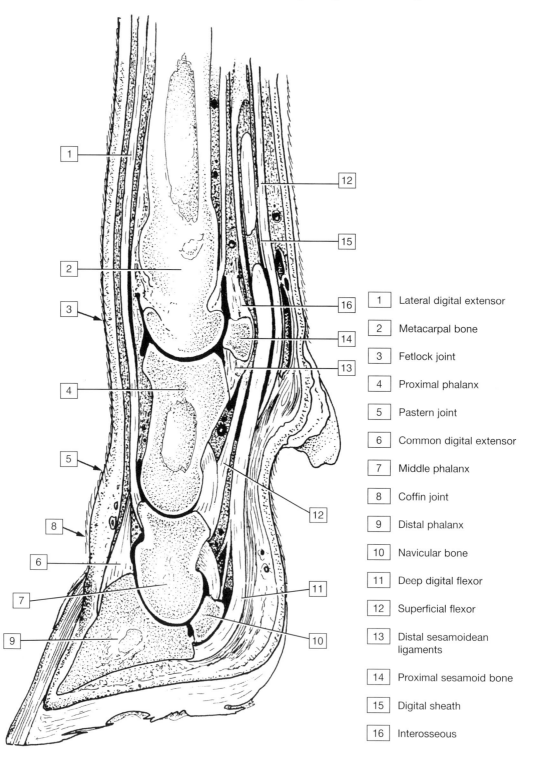

1	Lateral digital extensor
2	Metacarpal bone
3	Fetlock joint
4	Proximal phalanx
5	Pastern joint
6	Common digital extensor
7	Middle phalanx
8	Coffin joint
9	Distal phalanx
10	Navicular bone
11	Deep digital flexor
12	Superficial flexor
13	Distal sesamoidean ligaments
14	Proximal sesamoid bone
15	Digital sheath
16	Interosseous

FIGURE 6-31

Sagittal section of the medial digit of the bovine forefoot

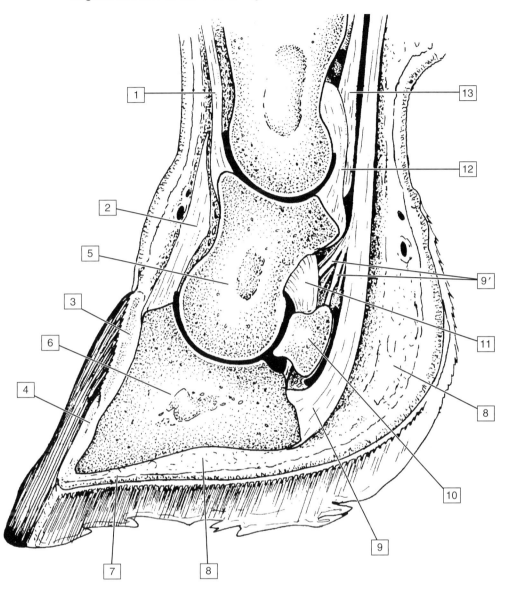

1	Proper (medial) digital extensor	
2	Common digital extensor	
3	Coronary dermis	
4	Laminar dermis	
5	Middle phalanx	
6	Distal phalanx	
7	Sole dermis covered by sole	
8	Digital cushion	

9	Deep digital flexor
9'	Fibers of deep digital flexor to the middle phalanx and navicular bone
10	Navicular bone
11	Collateral navicular ligament
12	Palmar ligaments of pastern joint
13	Superficial digital flexor

FIGURE 6-32

Dermis over which the horny bovine hoof
is produced, abaxial and ground surface

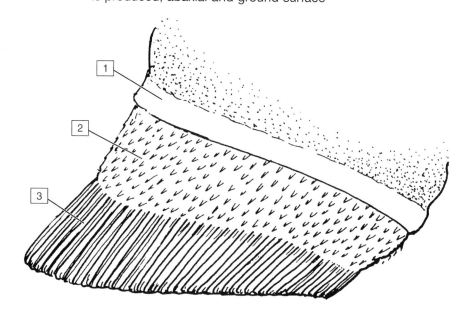

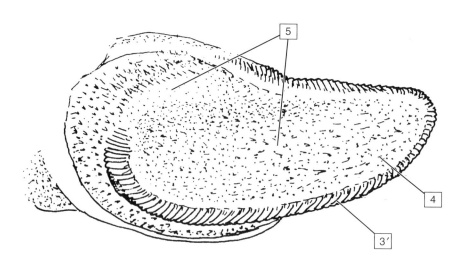

1	Perioplic dermis	3'	Terminal papillae at the distal ends of the laminae
2	Coronary dermis	4	Sole dermis
3	Laminar dermis	5	Dermis of the bulb

FIGURE 6-33   The Principal Veins of the Bovine Forelimb

A, Left foot, lateral view. *B*, Right foot, dorsal view.

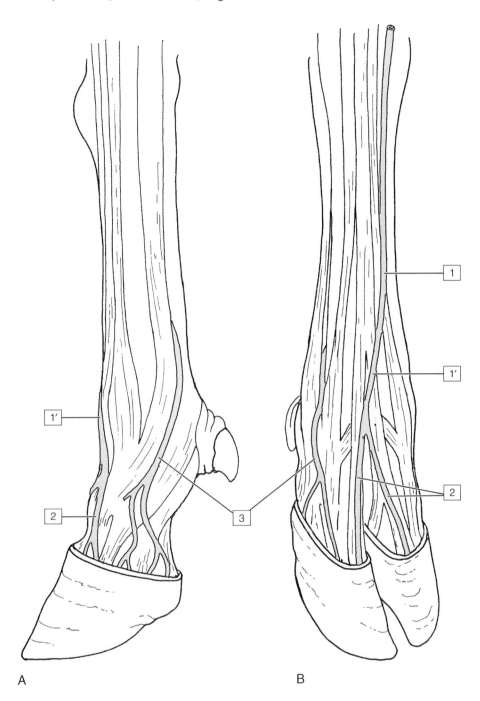

A

B

| 1 | Accessory cephalic v. | | 2 | Dorsal digital v. |
| 1' | Dorsal common digital v. III | | 3 | Abaxial palmar digital vv. |

FIGURE 6-34

The principal nerves of the bovine right forefoot in lateral and dorsal views

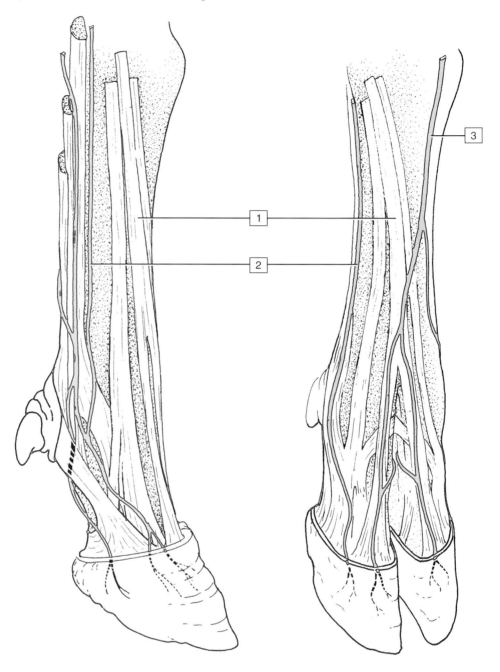

1	Digital extensor tendons	3	Superficial branch of radial n.
2	Dorsal branch of ulnar n.		

FIGURE 6-35   Left Porcine Forefoot, Caudomedial View

Inset shows the carpal glands on the undersurface of the skin, enlarged.

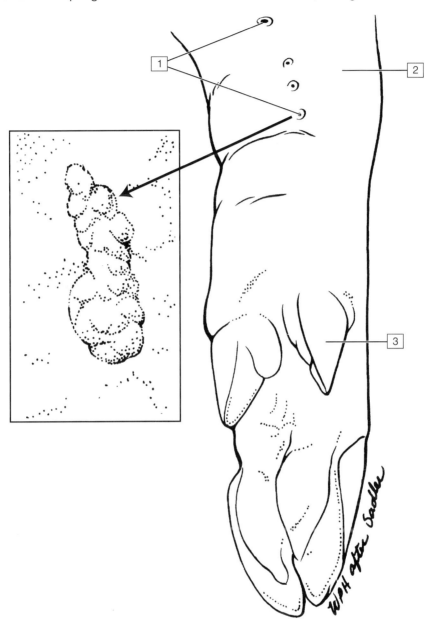

| 1 | Carpal glands | | 3 | Hoof of medial dewclaw |

| 2 | Medial surface of carpus |

FIGURE 6-36

Skeleton of avian left wing, partially extended laterally

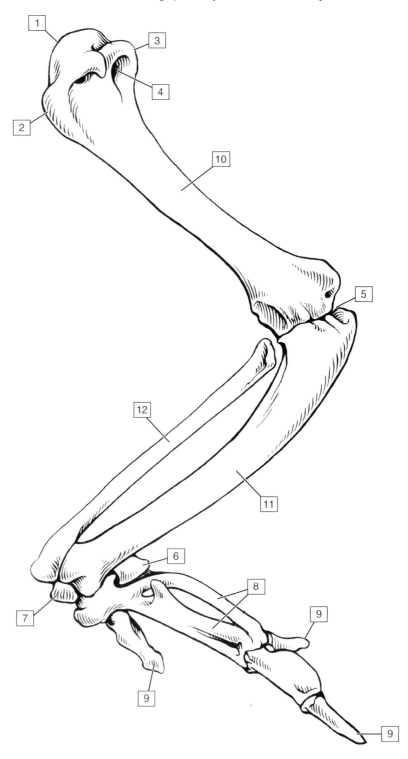

1	Head	4	Pneumatic foramen	7	Radial carpal	10	Humerus
2	Dorsal tubercle	5	Elbow joint	8	Carpometacarpals	11	Ulna
3	Ventral tubercle	6	Ulnar carpal	9	Digits	12	Radius

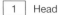

Saunders Veterinary Anatomy Coloring Book

FIGURE 6-37

Superficial dissection of laterally extended avian left wing, ventral surface

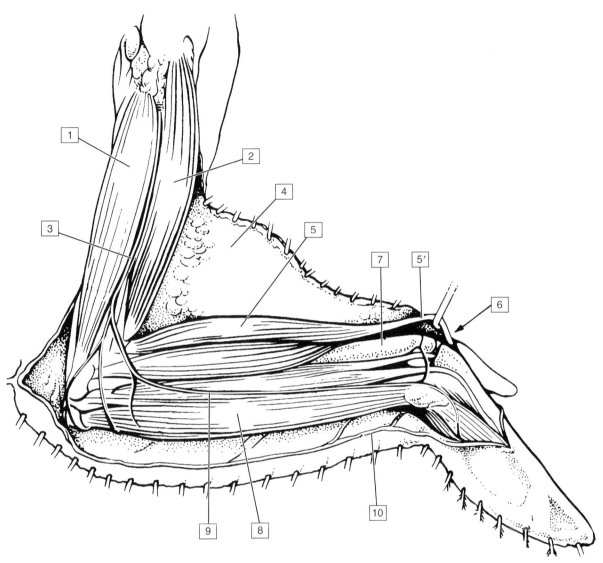

1 Triceps	6 Carpal joint
2 Biceps	7 Subcutaneous part of radius
3 Brachial vein	8 Flexor carpi ulnaris
4 Skin fold (propatagium)	9 Cutaneous ulnar (wing) vein
5 Extensor carpi radialis	10 Reflected skin
5' Tendon of extensor carpi radialis	

FIGURE 6-38 Bones of the Carpal Skeleton

Carnivores (*Car*), horse (*eq*), cattle (*bo*), and pig (*su*), schematic.
Roman numerals identify the metacarpal bones.

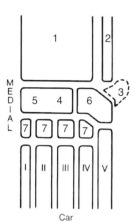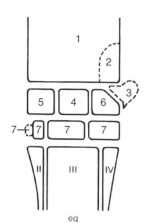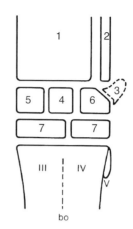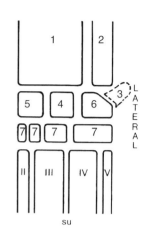

1	Radius	5	Radial carpal bone
2	Ulna	6	Ulnar carpal bone
3	Accessory carpal bone	7	Distal carpal bones
4	Intermediate carpal bone		

Saunders Veterinary Anatomy Coloring Book

FIGURE 6-39   Schematic Representation of Nail, Claw, and Hoof

A-C, Longitudinal section, palmer surface, and head-on view of human fingertip. *D, E,* Longitudinal section and palmer surface of canine claw. *F, G,* Longitudinal section and ground surface of equine hoof.

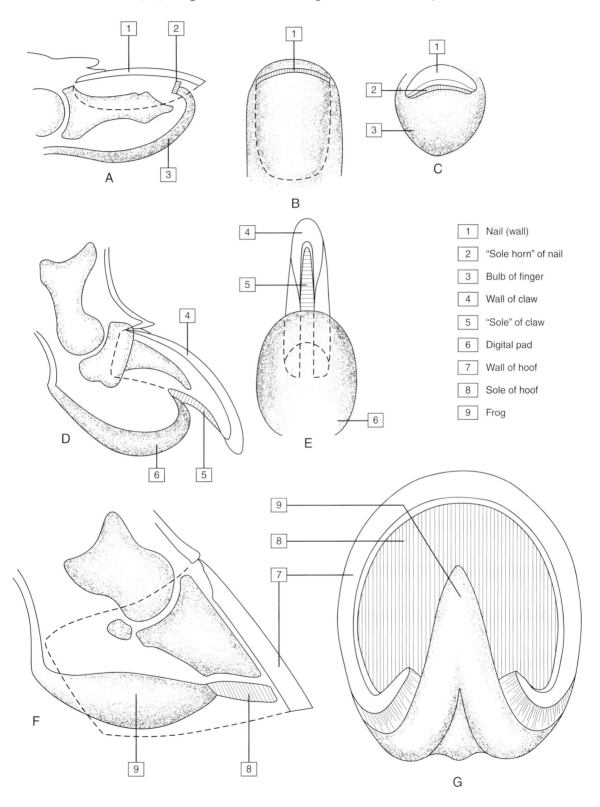

1	Nail (wall)
2	"Sole horn" of nail
3	Bulb of finger
4	Wall of claw
5	"Sole" of claw
6	Digital pad
7	Wall of hoof
8	Sole of hoof
9	Frog

7 THE HINDLIMB

FIGURE 7-1   Skeleton of Canine Right Pes, Dorsal View

Roman numerals identify the metatarsal bones.

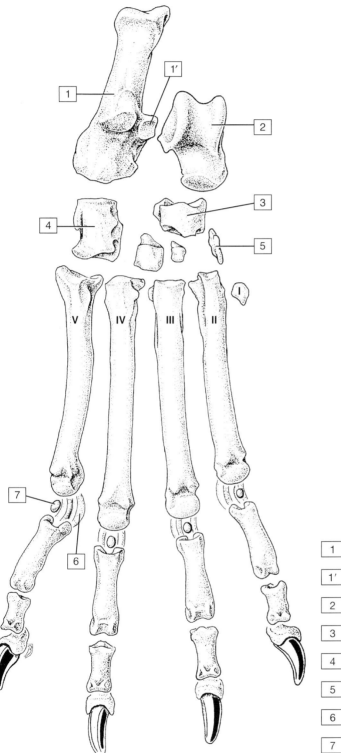

1	Calcaneus
1′	Sustentaculum tali
2	Talus
3	Central tarsal
4	Fourth tarsal
5	First, second, and third tarsal bones in distal row
6	Proximal sesamoid bones
7	Dorsal sesamoid bones

FIGURE 7-2   Canine Left Stifle Joint, Cranial Views (*A-C*)

The extent of the joint capsule is shown in *B*. The patella has been removed in *C*.

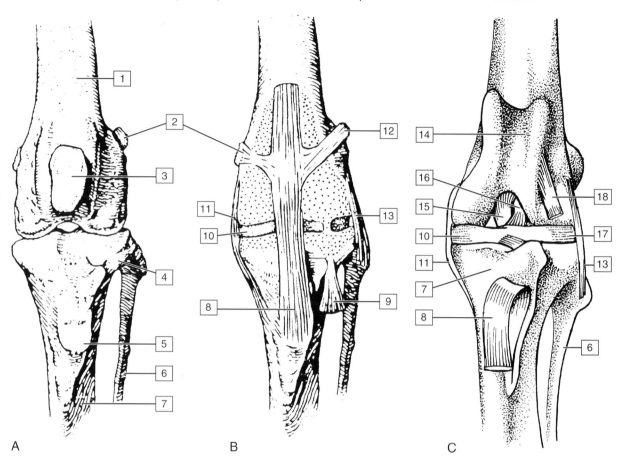

A   B   C

1	Femur		10	Medial meniscus
2	Sesamoids in gastrocnemius		11	Medial collateral ligament
3	Patella		12	Lateral femoropatellar ligament
4	Extensor groove		13	Lateral collateral ligament
5	Tibial tuberosity		14	Trochlea
6	Fibula		15	Caudal cruciate ligament
7	Tibia		16	Cranial cruciate ligament
8	Patellar ligament		17	Lateral meniscus
9	Tendon of long digital extensor passing through extensor groove		18	Stump of 9

FIGURE 7-3   Muscles of the Canine Hindquarter
and Thigh, Lateral (*A*) and Medial (*B*) Views

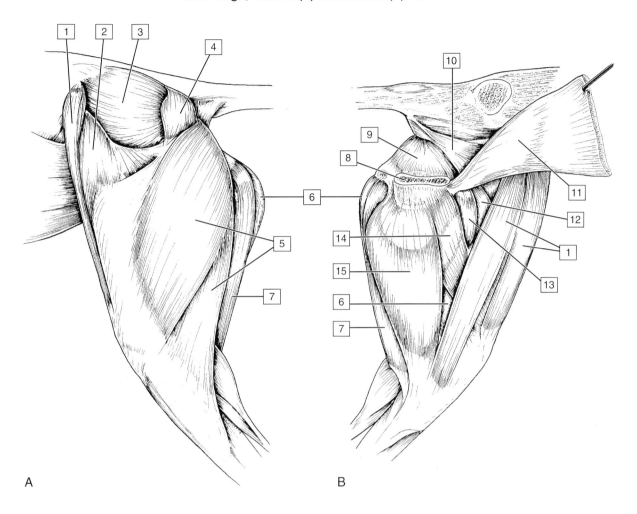

A

B

1	Sartorius	9	Internal obturator
2	Tensor fasciae latae	10	Levator ani
3	Gluteus medius	11	Rectus abdominis
4	Gluteus superficialis	12	Quadriceps (vastus medialis)
5	Biceps	13	Pectineus
6	Semimembranosus	14	Adductor
7	Semitendinosus	15	Gracilis
8	Pelvic symphysis		

FIGURE 7-4

Muscles of the left canine leg, lateral and medial views

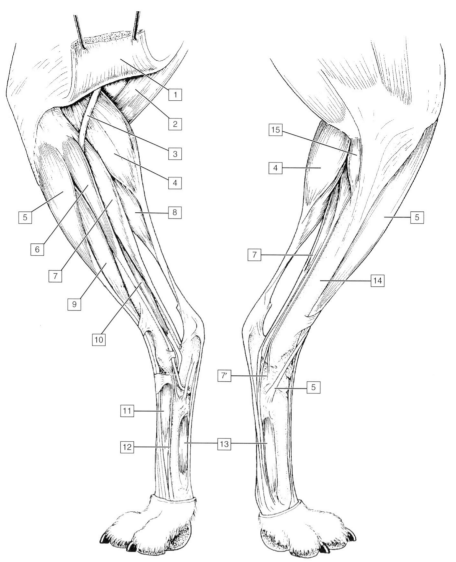

1	Biceps femoris
2	Semitendinosus
3	Peroneal nerve
4	Gastrocnemius
5	Tibialis cranialis
6	Peroneus longus
7	Lateral deep digital flexor
7′	Tendon of the smaller medial deep digital flexor
8	Superficial digital flexor
9	Long digital extensor
10	Peroneus brevis
11	Extensor brevis
12	Tendon of lateral digital extensor
13	Interossei
14	Tibia
15	Popliteus

Saunders Veterinary Anatomy Coloring Book

FIGURE 7-5

Transverse section of the canine left thigh

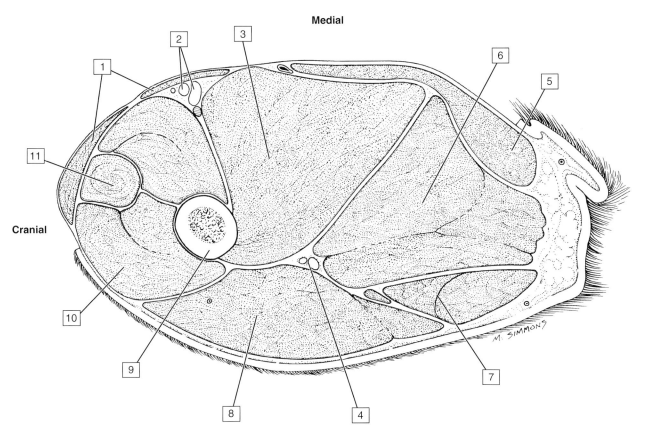

Medial

Cranial

M. SIMMONS

1	Sartorius		7	Semitendinosus
2	Femoral vessels		8	Biceps femoris
3	Adductor		9	Femur
4	Sciatic nerve		10	Vastus lateralis (of quadriceps)
5	Gracilis		11	Rectus femoris
6	Semimembranosus			

FIGURE 7-6   Canine Left Hindlimb

The inset shows the actual appearance
of the lateral saphenous vein, lateral view.

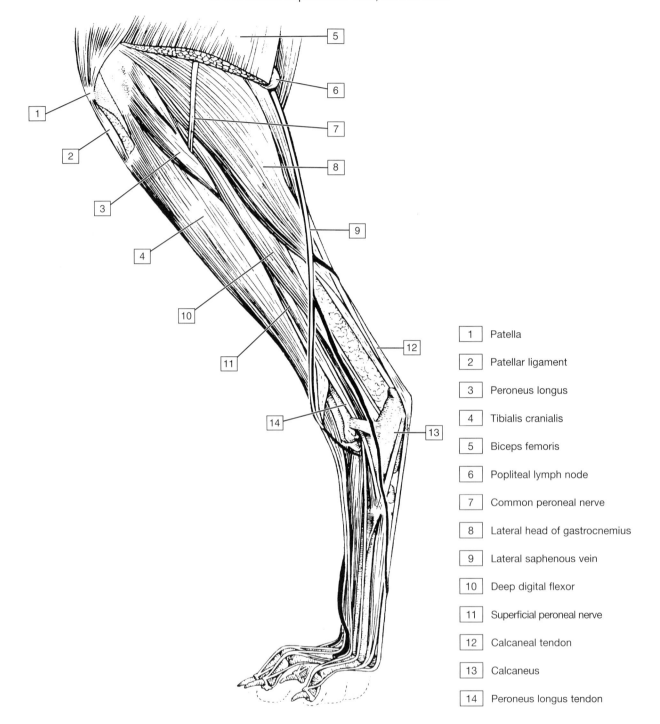

1	Patella
2	Patellar ligament
3	Peroneus longus
4	Tibialis cranialis
5	Biceps femoris
6	Popliteal lymph node
7	Common peroneal nerve
8	Lateral head of gastrocnemius
9	Lateral saphenous vein
10	Deep digital flexor
11	Superficial peroneal nerve
12	Calcaneal tendon
13	Calcaneus
14	Peroneus longus tendon

FIGURE 7-7

Superficial muscles of the canine left pelvic limb, medial view

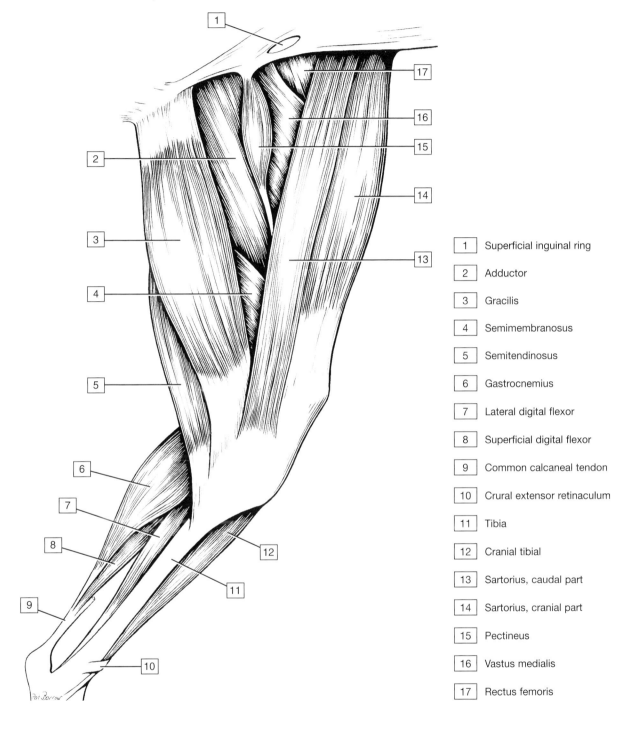

1	Superficial inguinal ring
2	Adductor
3	Gracilis
4	Semimembranosus
5	Semitendinosus
6	Gastrocnemius
7	Lateral digital flexor
8	Superficial digital flexor
9	Common calcaneal tendon
10	Crural extensor retinaculum
11	Tibia
12	Cranial tibial
13	Sartorius, caudal part
14	Sartorius, cranial part
15	Pectineus
16	Vastus medialis
17	Rectus femoris

FIGURE 7-8

Muscle attachments on the canine pelvis and left pelvic limb, medial view

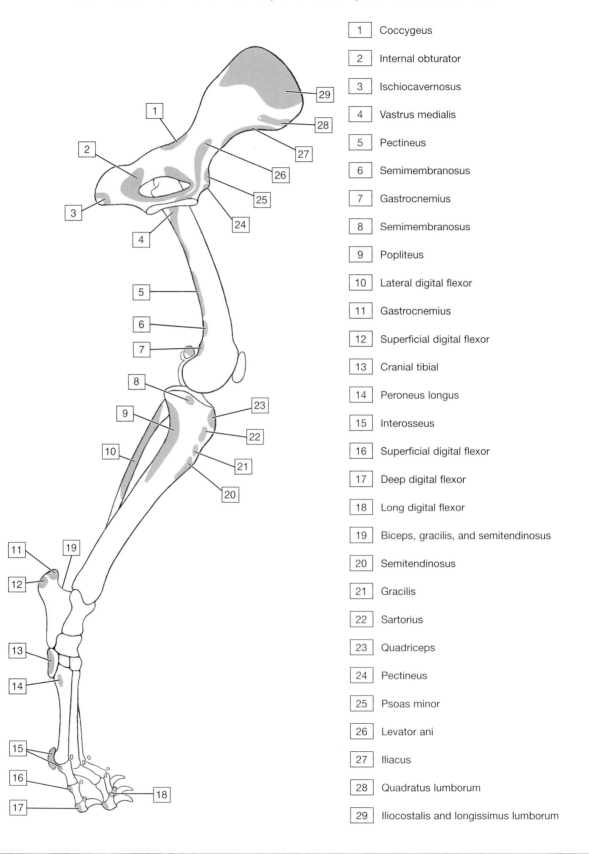

1	Coccygeus
2	Internal obturator
3	Ischiocavernosus
4	Vastrus medialis
5	Pectineus
6	Semimembranosus
7	Gastrocnemius
8	Semimembranosus
9	Popliteus
10	Lateral digital flexor
11	Gastrocnemius
12	Superficial digital flexor
13	Cranial tibial
14	Peroneus longus
15	Interosseus
16	Superficial digital flexor
17	Deep digital flexor
18	Long digital flexor
19	Biceps, gracilis, and semitendinosus
20	Semitendinosus
21	Gracilis
22	Sartorius
23	Quadriceps
24	Pectineus
25	Psoas minor
26	Levator ani
27	Iliacus
28	Quadratus lumborum
29	Iliocostalis and longissimus lumborum

FIGURE 7-9

Arteries of the canine right pelvic limb, schematic medial view

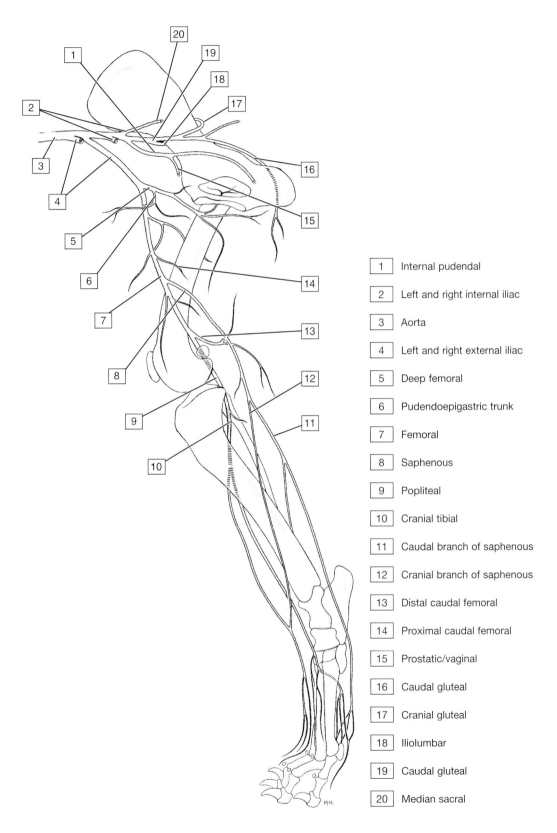

1	Internal pudendal
2	Left and right internal iliac
3	Aorta
4	Left and right external iliac
5	Deep femoral
6	Pudendoepigastric trunk
7	Femoral
8	Saphenous
9	Popliteal
10	Cranial tibial
11	Caudal branch of saphenous
12	Cranial branch of saphenous
13	Distal caudal femoral
14	Proximal caudal femoral
15	Prostatic/vaginal
16	Caudal gluteal
17	Cranial gluteal
18	Iliolumbar
19	Caudal gluteal
20	Median sacral

FIGURE 7-10

Arteries and nerves of the canine right thigh and crus, lateral view

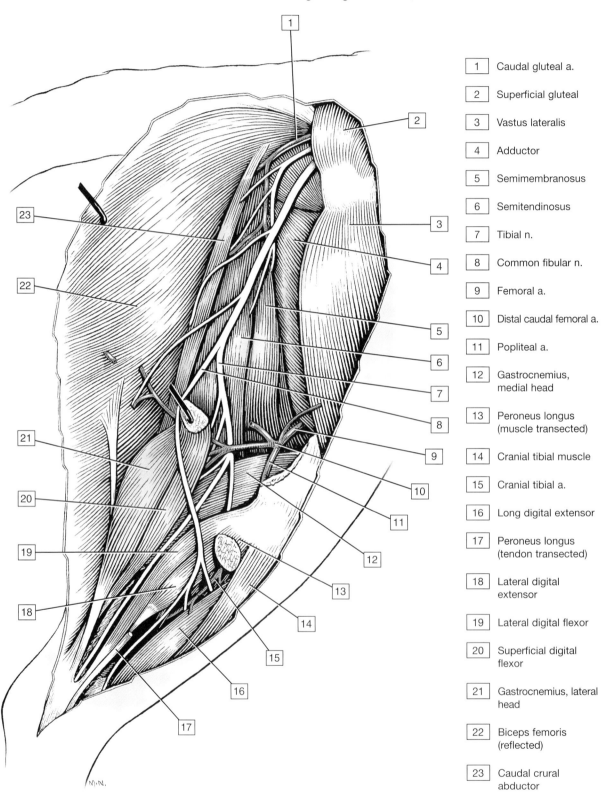

1	Caudal gluteal a.
2	Superficial gluteal
3	Vastus lateralis
4	Adductor
5	Semimembranosus
6	Semitendinosus
7	Tibial n.
8	Common fibular n.
9	Femoral a.
10	Distal caudal femoral a.
11	Popliteal a.
12	Gastrocnemius, medial head
13	Peroneus longus (muscle transected)
14	Cranial tibial muscle
15	Cranial tibial a.
16	Long digital extensor
17	Peroneus longus (tendon transected)
18	Lateral digital extensor
19	Lateral digital flexor
20	Superficial digital flexor
21	Gastrocnemius, lateral head
22	Biceps femoris (reflected)
23	Caudal crural abductor

FIGURE 7-11

Cranial and lateral views of equine left femur

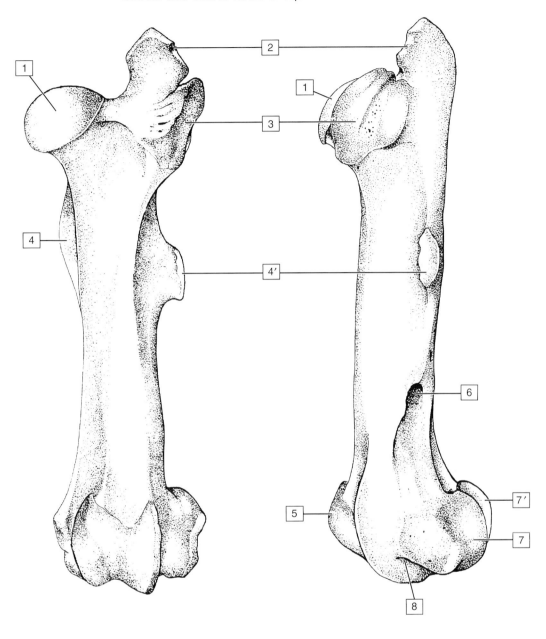

1	Head		5	Enlarged proximal end of medial trochlear ridge
2	Cranial part of greater trochanter		6	Supracondylar fossa
3	Caudal part of greater trochanter		7	Lateral condyle
4	Lesser trochanter		7′	Medial condyle
4′	Third trochanter		8	Extensor fossa

FIGURE 7-12

Cranial and lateral views of equine left tibia and fibula

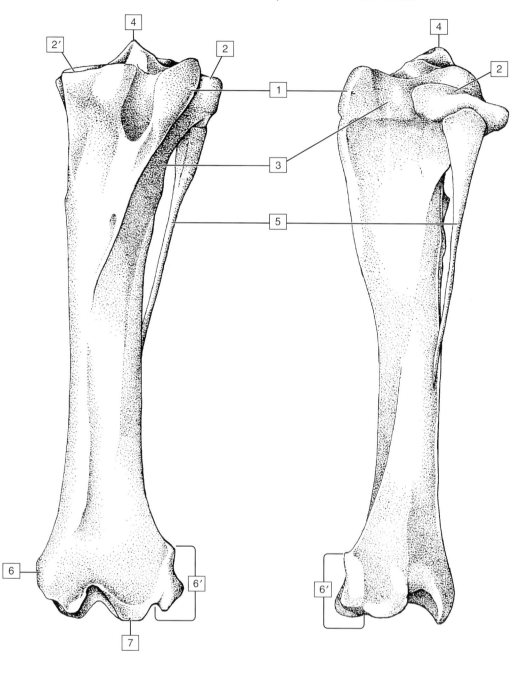

1	Tibial tuberosity
2	Lateral condyle
2'	Medial condyle
3	Extensor groove
4	Intercondylar eminence

5	Fibula
6	Medial malleolus
6'	Lateral malleolus in the horse (representing distal end of fibula)
7	Cochlea

FIGURE 7-13

Skeleton of the equine left hindlimb, lateral view

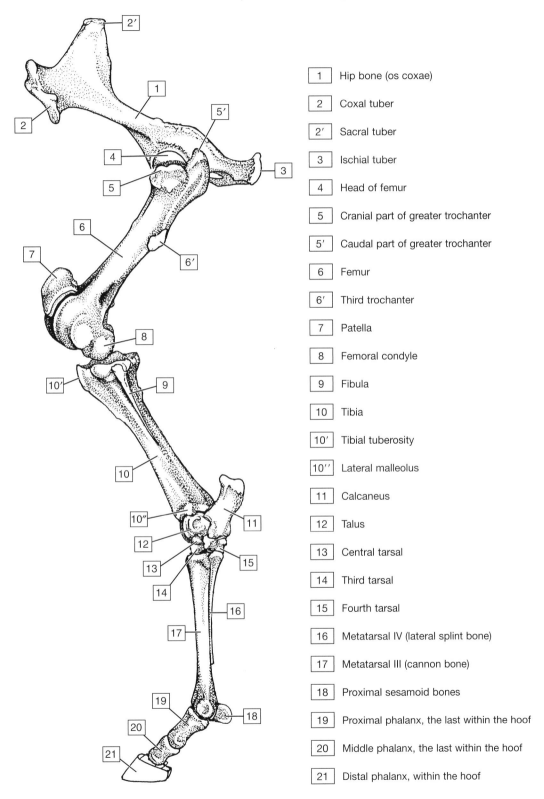

1	Hip bone (os coxae)
2	Coxal tuber
2′	Sacral tuber
3	Ischial tuber
4	Head of femur
5	Cranial part of greater trochanter
5′	Caudal part of greater trochanter
6	Femur
6′	Third trochanter
7	Patella
8	Femoral condyle
9	Fibula
10	Tibia
10′	Tibial tuberosity
10′′	Lateral malleolus
11	Calcaneus
12	Talus
13	Central tarsal
14	Third tarsal
15	Fourth tarsal
16	Metatarsal IV (lateral splint bone)
17	Metatarsal III (cannon bone)
18	Proximal sesamoid bones
19	Proximal phalanx, the last within the hoof
20	Middle phalanx, the last within the hoof
21	Distal phalanx, within the hoof

FIGURE 7-14

Muscles of the equine thigh, medial view

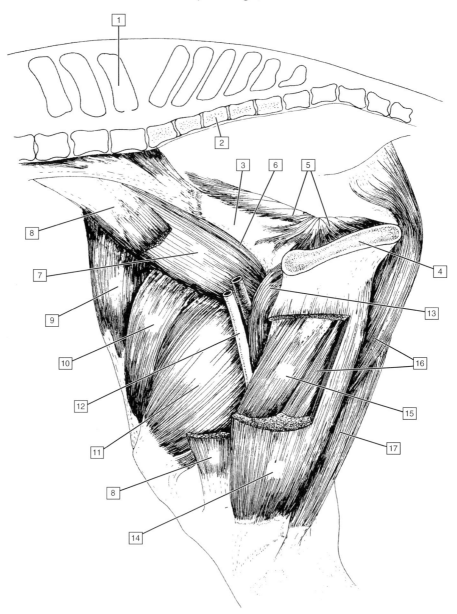

1	Last lumbar vertebra	6	Psoas minor	
2	Sacrum	7	Iliopsoas	
3	Shaft of ilium	8	Sartorius, resected	
4	Pelvic symphysis	9	Tensor fasciae latae	
5	Internal obturator			

10	Rectus femoris
11	Vastus medialis
12	Femoral vessels in femoral triangle
13	Pectineus

14	Gracilis, fenestrated
15	Adductor
16	Semimembranosus
17	Semitendinosus

Name the nerve that supplies 13, 14, and 15.

FIGURE 7-15

Equine left stifle joint, cranial view

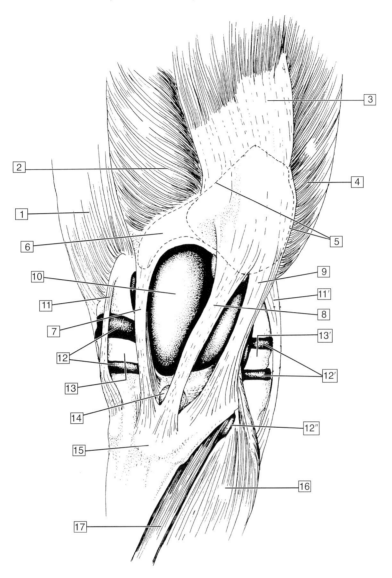

1	Adductor	7	Medial patellar ligament	11'	Lateral collateral ligaments
2	Vastus medialis	8	Intermediate patellar ligament	12	Medial femorotibial joint capsule
3	Rectus femoris	9	Lateral patellar ligament	12'	Lateral femorotibial joint capsule
4	Vastus lateralis	10	Joint capsule over medial ridge of femoral trochlea	12''	Recess of 12' under combined tendon of peroneus tertius and long digital extensor
5	Outline of patella	11	Medial collateral ligament		
6	Outline of patellar fibrocartilage				

13	Medial meniscus
13'	Lateral menisci
14	Distal infrapatellar bursa
15	Tibial tuberosity
16	Long digital extensor
17	Tibialis cranialis

Name the nerve that supplies 2, 3, and 4.

FIGURE 7-16 Bursae, Tendon Sheaths,
and Joint Pouches of the Equine Left Hock

Proximal surface of a transection.

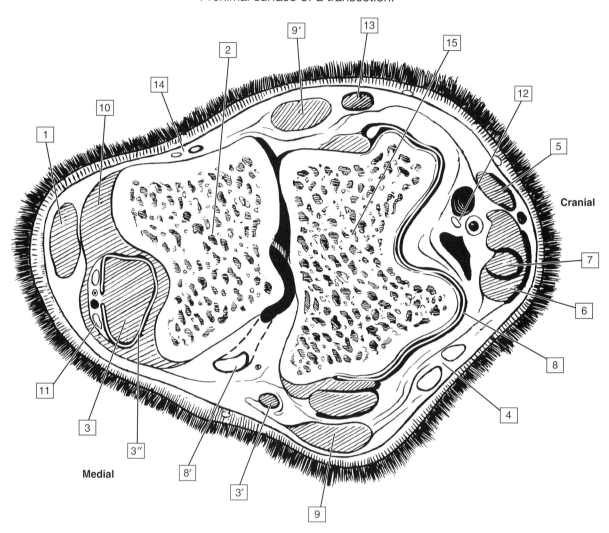

1	Superficial digital flexor		8'	Medioplantar pouch of tarsocrural joint
2	Calcaneus		9	Medial collateral ligament (superficial part)
3	Lateral deep digital flexor and tibialis caudalis		9'	Lateral collateral ligament (superficial part)
3'	Tendon of medial deep digital flexor		10	Long plantar ligament
3''	Tarsal sheath		11	Plantar nerves and saphenous vessels
4	Cranial branch of medial saphenous vein		12	Cranial tibial vessels and deep peroneal nerve
5	Long digital extensor		13	Lateral digital extensor
6	Peroneus tertius		14	Caudal cutaneous sural nerve and lateral saphenous vein
7	Tibialis cranialis		15	Talus
8	Dorsal and medioplantar pouches of tarsocrural joint			

FIGURE 7-17

Principal arteries of the equine right hindlimb, caudal view

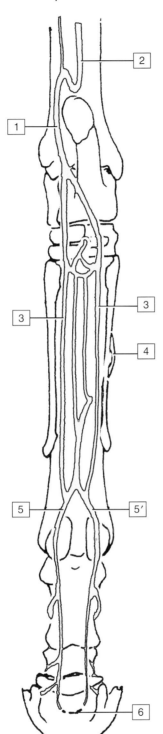

1	Saphenous a.
2	Caudal tibial a.
3	Medial plantar aa.
4	Dorsal metatarsal a.
5	Medial digital a.
5′	Lateral digital a.
6	Terminal arch, anastomosis of digital arteries within the distal phalanx

FIGURE 7-18

Nerves of the equine right hindfoot

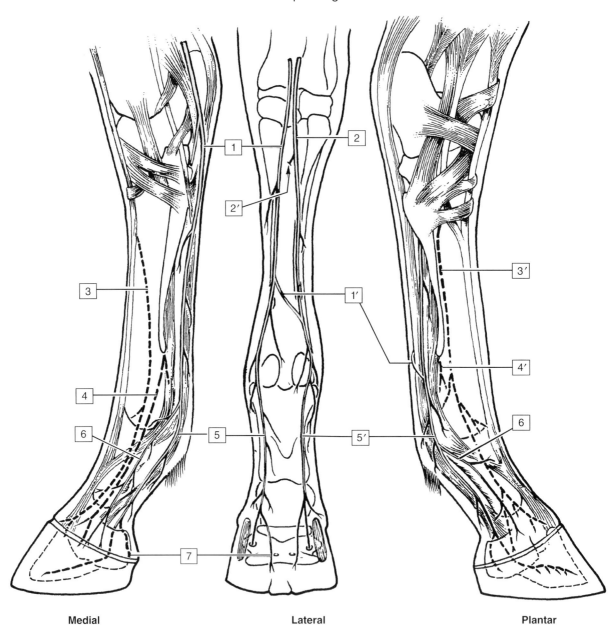

Medial   Lateral   Plantar

1	Medial plantar n. (from tibial)	4	Medial plantar metatarsal n. (from lateral plantar)
1'	Communicating branch	4'	Lateral plantar metatarsal n. (from lateral plantar)
2	Lateral plantar n. (from tibial)	5	Medial digital n.
2'	Deep branch (for plantar metatarsal nn.), cut	5'	Lateral digital n.
3	Medial dorsal metatarsal n. (from deep peroneal)	6	Dorsal branch of digital n.
3'	Lateral dorsal metatarsal n. (from deep peroneal)	7	Branch to digital cushion

FIGURE 7-19

Bovine sacrosciatic ligament, left lateral view

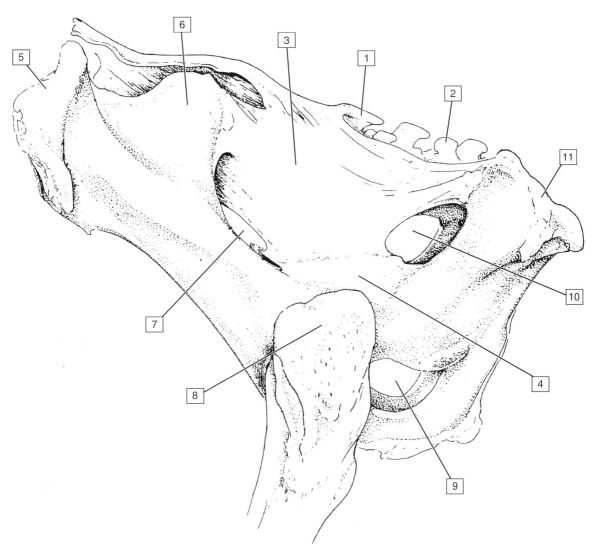

1	Sacrum	7	Greater sciatic foramen
2	Caudal vertebra(e)	8	Greater trochanter
3	Sacrotuberous ligament	9	Obturator foramen
4	Ischial spine	10	Lesser sciatic foramen
5	Coxal tuber	11	Ischial tube
6	Sacral tuber		

FIGURE 7-20

Muscles of the bovine left hindlimb, lateral view

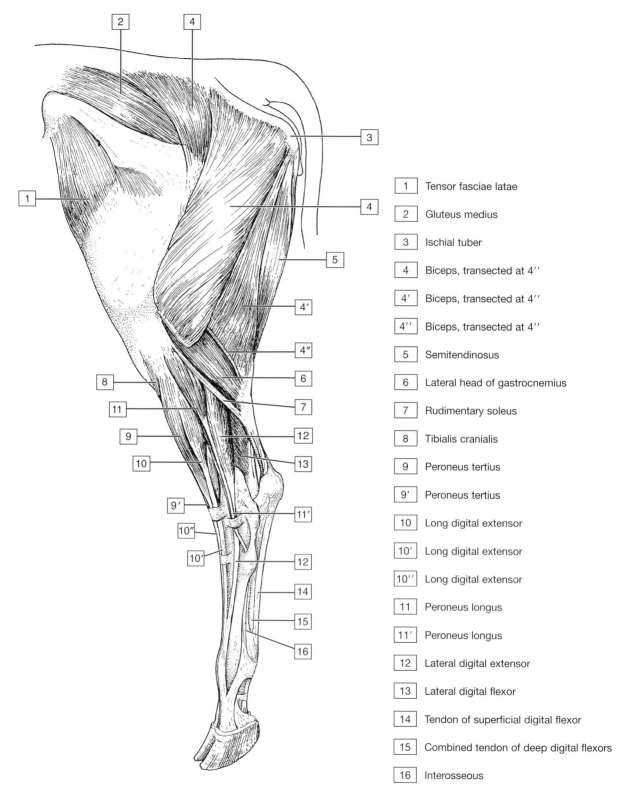

1	Tensor fasciae latae
2	Gluteus medius
3	Ischial tuber
4	Biceps, transected at 4''
4'	Biceps, transected at 4''
4''	Biceps, transected at 4''
5	Semitendinosus
6	Lateral head of gastrocnemius
7	Rudimentary soleus
8	Tibialis cranialis
9	Peroneus tertius
9'	Peroneus tertius
10	Long digital extensor
10'	Long digital extensor
10''	Long digital extensor
11	Peroneus longus
11'	Peroneus longus
12	Lateral digital extensor
13	Lateral digital flexor
14	Tendon of superficial digital flexor
15	Combined tendon of deep digital flexors
16	Interosseous

FIGURE 7-21

Transverse section of the bovine left leg

Medial

Cranial

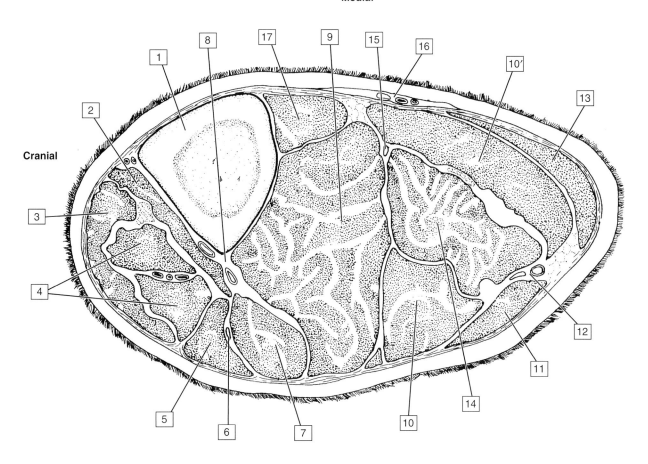

1	Tibia
2	Tibialis cranialis
3	Peroneus tertius
4	Long digital extensor
5	Peroneus longus
6	Peroneal nerve
7	Lateral digital extensor
8	Cranial tibial vessels
9	Deep digital flexors
10	Lateral head gastrocnemius

10′	Medial head of gastrocnemius
11	Biceps femoris
12	Caudal cutaneous sural nerve and lateral saphenous vein
13	Semitendinosus
14	Superficial digital flexor
15	Tibial nerve
16	Saphenous vessels and nerve
17	Popliteus

FIGURE 7-22   The Major Veins of the Bovine Hindlimb

A, Right hindfoot, dorsolateral view. *B,* Left hind foot, dorsomedial view.

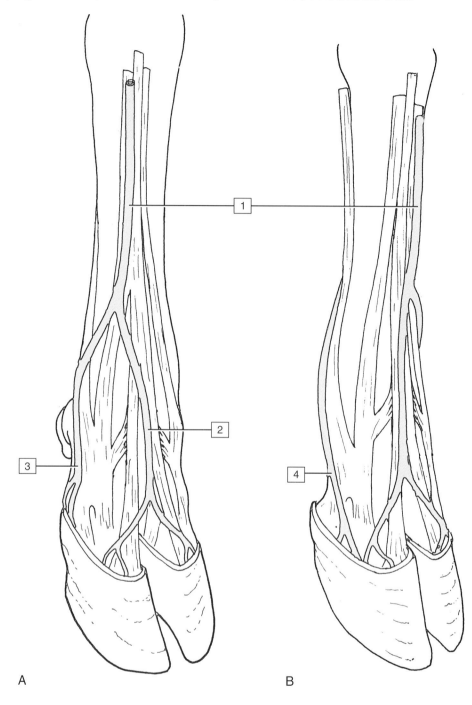

A

B

| 1 | Cranial tributary of lateral saphenous v. |
| 2 | Dorsal common digital v. III |

| 3 | Plantar v. of lateral digit |
| 4 | Plantar v. of medial digits |

FIGURE 7-23   Nerves of the Right Bovine Hindlimb

A, Right hind foot, dorsolateral view. *B,* Right hind foot, plantar view.

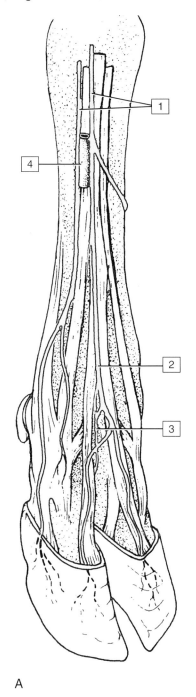

A

B

1	Lateral and middle branches of superficial peroneal n.	4	Cranial tributary of lateral saphenous vein
2	Dorsal common digital n. III	5	Medial and lateral plantar nn.
3	Deep peroneal n.	6	Plantar common digital n. III

FIGURE 7-24

Transverse section of the bovine left cannon

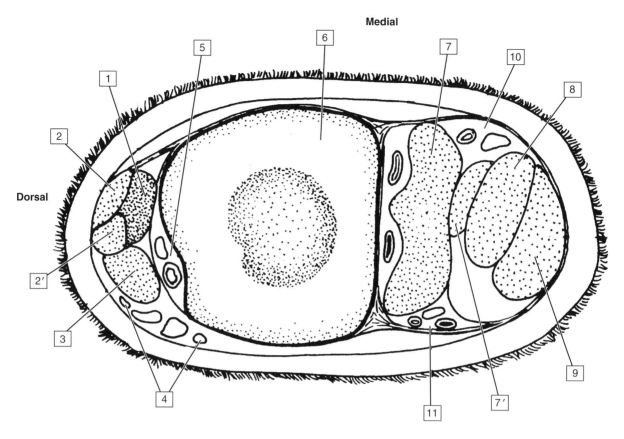

1	Extensor brevis
2	Long digital extensor
2′	Long digital extensor
3	Lateral digital extensor
4	Branches of superficial peroneal nerve and cranial tributary of lateral saphenous vein
5	Deep peroneal nerve and dorsal metatarsal artery (continuation of cranial tibial)

6	Metatarsal bone
7	Interosseous
7′	Band from interosseous to superficial digital flexor
8	Deep digital flexor
9	Superficial digital flexor
10	Medial plantar nerve and vessel
11	Lateral plantar nerve and vessel

FIGURE 7-25

Lymph flow of the porcine hindlimb, lateral view

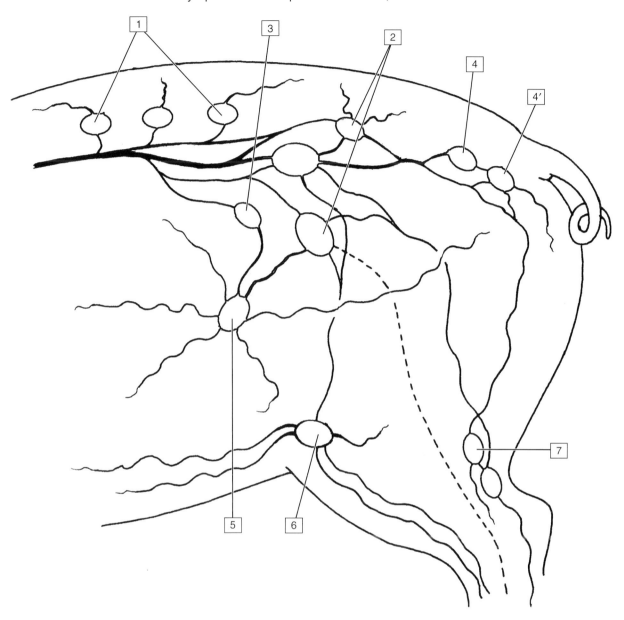

1	Lumbar aortic nodes	4'	Gluteal nodes
2	Medial iliac nodes	5	Subiliac nodes
3	Lateral iliac node	6	Superficial inguinal nodes
4	Ischial node	7	Popliteal nodes

FIGURE 7-26   Bones of the Tarsal Skeleton

Carnivores (*car*), horse (*eq*), cattle (*bo*), and pig (*su*), schematic.
Roman numerals identify the metatarsal bones. Arabic
numerals identify the distal tarsal bones.

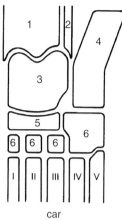
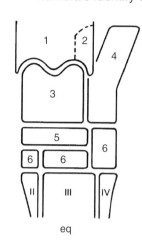
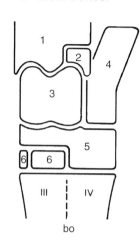
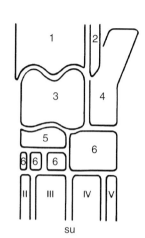

car

eq

bo

su

1	Radius	4	Calcaneus
2	Fibula	5	Central tarsal bone
3	Talus	6	Distal tarsal bones

EXOTICS

FIGURE 8-1

Musteline: skeletal anatomy of a ferret

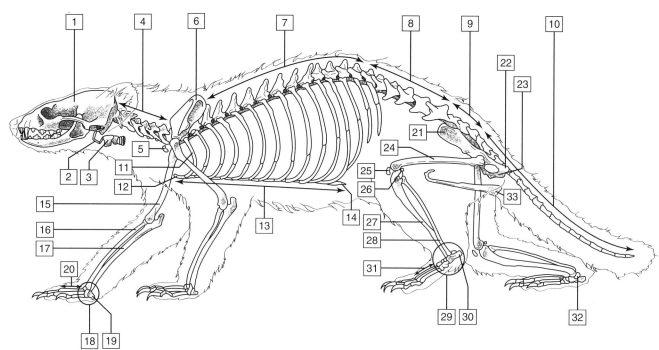

1 Calvaria	10 Eighteen caudal vertebrae	19 Accessory carpal bone	28 Fibula
2 Hyoid apparatus	11 First rib	20 Metacarpal bones	29 Tarsal bones
3 Larynx	12 Manubrium	21 Ilium	30 Calcaneus
4 Seven cervical vertebrae	13 Sternum	22 Ischium	31 Metatarsal bones
5 Clavicle	14 Xiphoid process	23 Pubis	32 Talus
6 Scapula	15 Humerus	24 Femur	33 Os penis
7 Fifteen thoracic vertebrae	16 Radius	25 Patella	
8 Five lumbar vertebrae	17 Ulna	26 Fabella	
9 Three sacral vertebrae	18 Carpal bones	27 Tibia	

FIGURE 8-2

Musteline: ventral view of the internal anatomy of a ferret

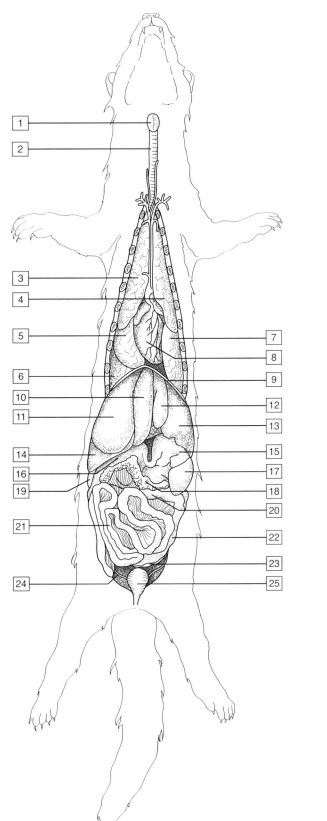

1	Larynx
2	Trachea
3	Right cranial lobe of lung
4	Left cranial lobe of lung
5	Right middle lobe of lung
6	Right caudal lobe of lung
7	Left caudal lobe of lung
8	Heart
9	Diaphragm
10	Quadrate lobe of liver
11	Right medial lobe of liver
12	Left medial lobe of liver
13	Left lateral lobe of liver
14	Right lateral lobe of liver
15	Stomach
16	Right kidney
17	Spleen
18	Pancreas
19	Duodenum
20	Transverse colon
21	Jejunoileum
22	Descending colon
23	Uterus
24	Ureter
25	Urinary bladder

Saunders Veterinary Anatomy Coloring Book

FIGURE 8-3

Leporine: skeletal anatomy of a rabbit

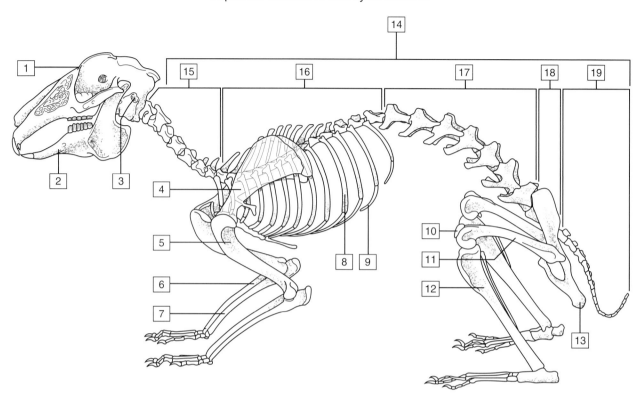

1	Skull	6	Radius	11	Femur	16	Thoracic
2	Mandible	7	Ulna	12	Tibia	17	Lumbar
3	Tympanic bulla	8	Rib	13	Pelvis	18	Sacral
4	Scapula	9	Cartilage	14	Vertebrae	19	Coccygeal
5	Humerus	10	Patella	15	Cervical		

Saunders Veterinary Anatomy Coloring Book

FIGURE 8-4

Leporine: ventral aspect of the internal anatomy of a female rabbit

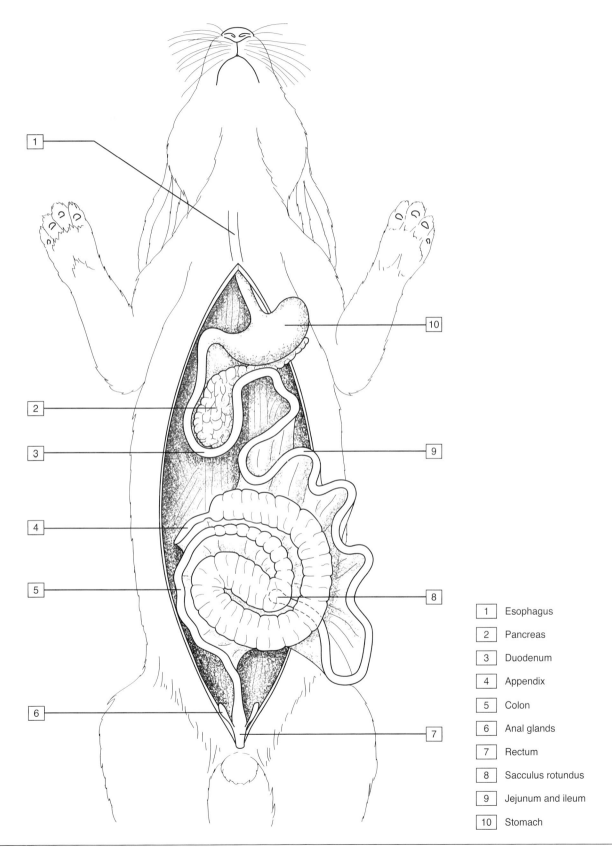

1	Esophagus
2	Pancreas
3	Duodenum
4	Appendix
5	Colon
6	Anal glands
7	Rectum
8	Sacculus rotundus
9	Jejunum and ileum
10	Stomach

FIGURE 8-5

Leporine: cross-section of skull showing dentition of
mandible and maxilla and of an individual tooth in a rabbit

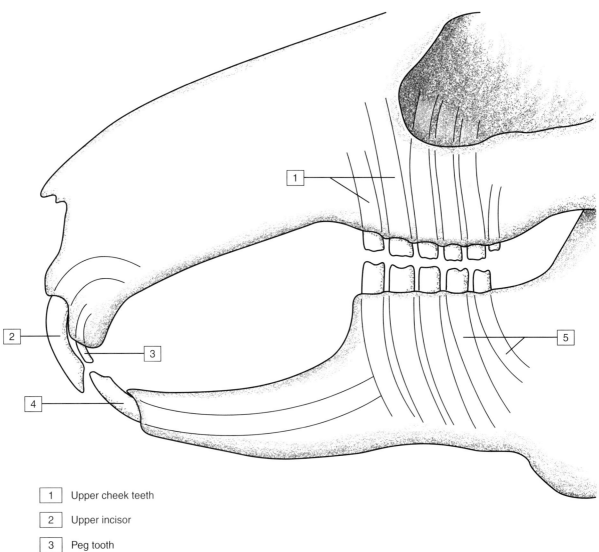

1	Upper cheek teeth
2	Upper incisor
3	Peg tooth
4	Lower incisor
5	Lower cheek teeth

Saunders Veterinary Anatomy Coloring Book

FIGURE 8-6

Leporine: vagina of a rabbit

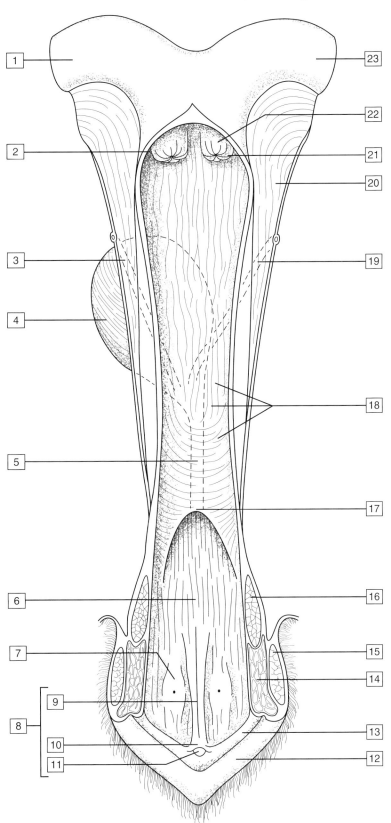

1	Left uterine horn
2	Vaginal fornix
3	Left ureter
4	Urinary bladder
5	Urethra
6	Vaginal vestibule
7	Greater vestibular gland
8	Clitoris
9	Corpus
10	Preputium
11	Glans
12	Greater lip of pudenda
13	Lesser lip of pudenda
14	Constrictor muscle of vestibule
15	Preputial gland
16	Vestibular bulb
17	External urethral opening
18	Vagina (ventral floor)
19	Right ureter
20	Uterine broad ligament
21	External uterine ostium
22	Right vaginal cervix
23	Right uterine horn

FIGURE 8-7

Cavine: ventral aspect of the internal anatomy of a female guinea pig

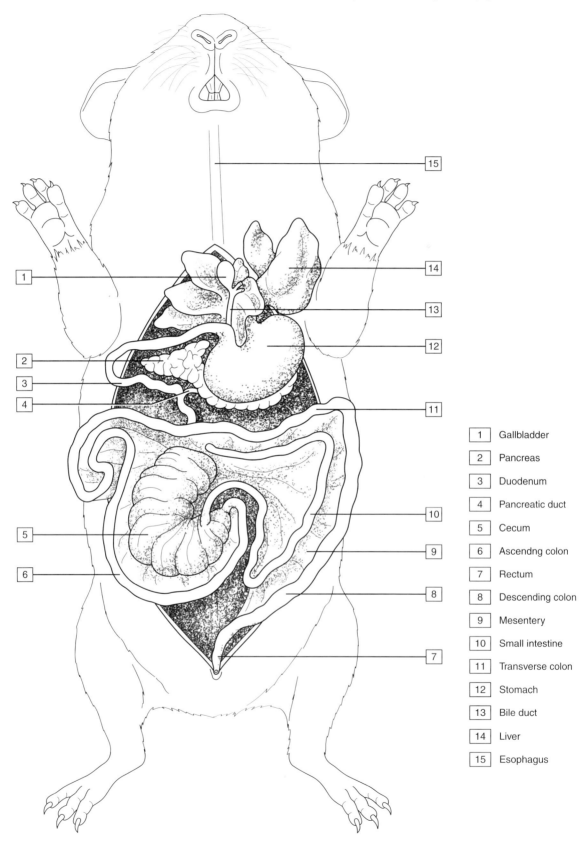

1	Gallbladder
2	Pancreas
3	Duodenum
4	Pancreatic duct
5	Cecum
6	Ascendng colon
7	Rectum
8	Descending colon
9	Mesentery
10	Small intestine
11	Transverse colon
12	Stomach
13	Bile duct
14	Liver
15	Esophagus

FIGURE 8-8

Cricetine: ventral aspect of the internal anatomy of a female hamster

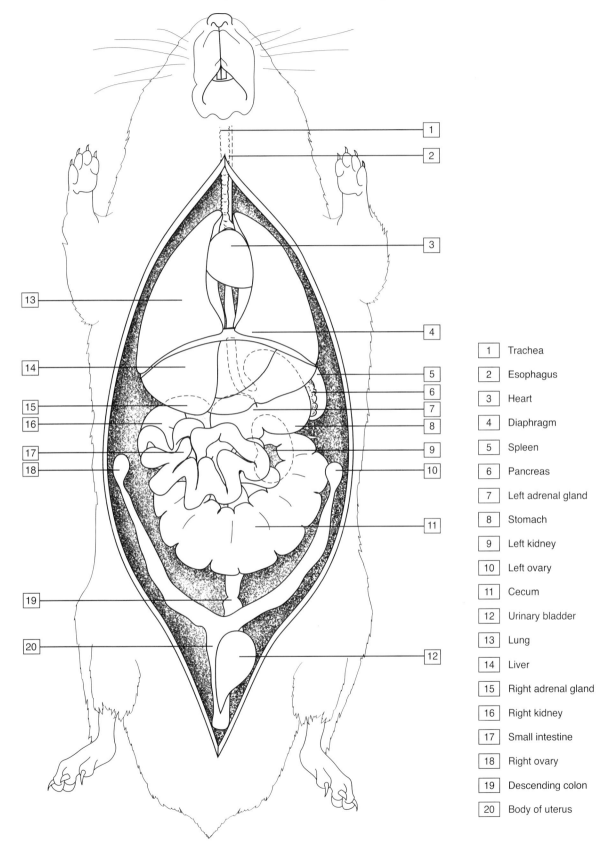

1	Trachea
2	Esophagus
3	Heart
4	Diaphragm
5	Spleen
6	Pancreas
7	Left adrenal gland
8	Stomach
9	Left kidney
10	Left ovary
11	Cecum
12	Urinary bladder
13	Lung
14	Liver
15	Right adrenal gland
16	Right kidney
17	Small intestine
18	Right ovary
19	Descending colon
20	Body of uterus

FIGURE 8-9

Cricetine: ventral aspect of the internal anatomy of a male Mongolian gerbil

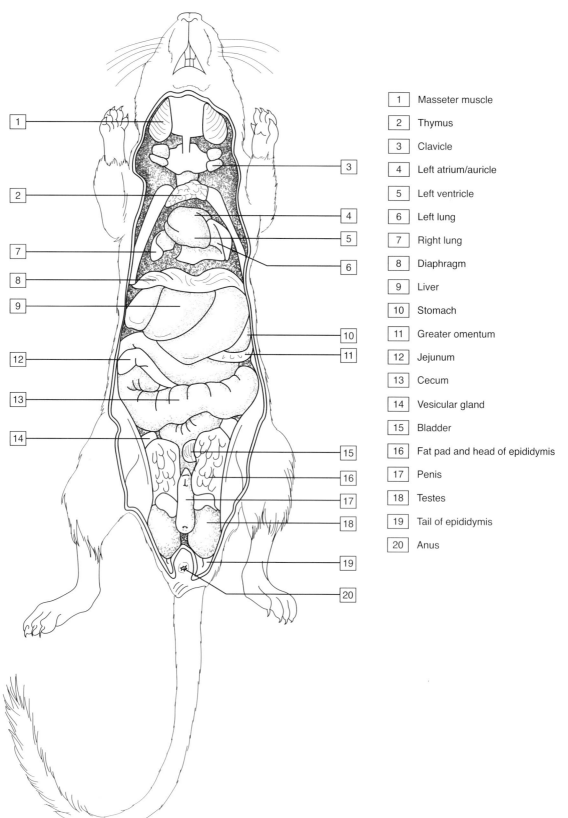

1	Masseter muscle
2	Thymus
3	Clavicle
4	Left atrium/auricle
5	Left ventricle
6	Left lung
7	Right lung
8	Diaphragm
9	Liver
10	Stomach
11	Greater omentum
12	Jejunum
13	Cecum
14	Vesicular gland
15	Bladder
16	Fat pad and head of epididymis
17	Penis
18	Testes
19	Tail of epididymis
20	Anus

Saunders Veterinary Anatomy Coloring Book

FIGURE 8-10

Erinaceidae: *Top,* Ventral aspect of the internal anatomy of a female African hedgehog. *Bottom,* Muscles used for curling body and spinal control

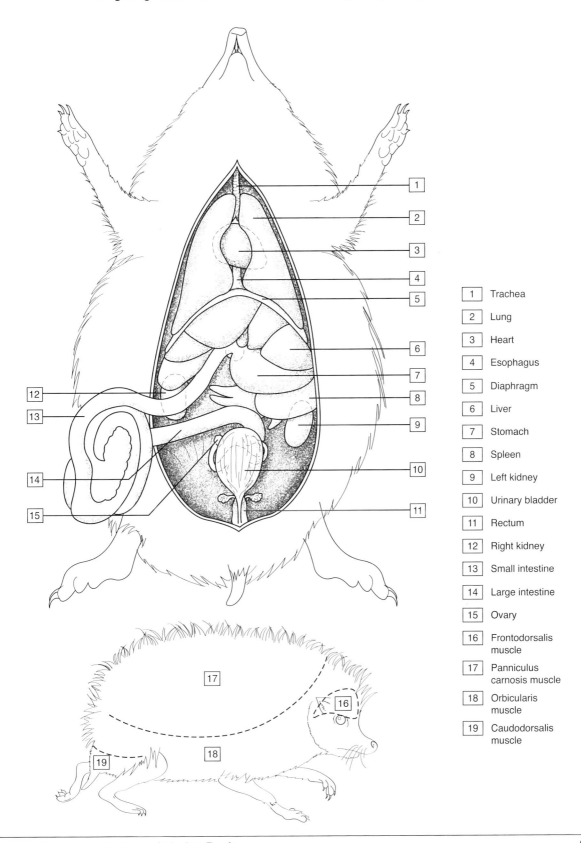

1	Trachea
2	Lung
3	Heart
4	Esophagus
5	Diaphragm
6	Liver
7	Stomach
8	Spleen
9	Left kidney
10	Urinary bladder
11	Rectum
12	Right kidney
13	Small intestine
14	Large intestine
15	Ovary
16	Frontodorsalis muscle
17	Panniculus carnosis muscle
18	Orbicularis muscle
19	Caudodorsalis muscle

FIGURE 8-11

Murine: ventral view of the internal anatomy of a female rat

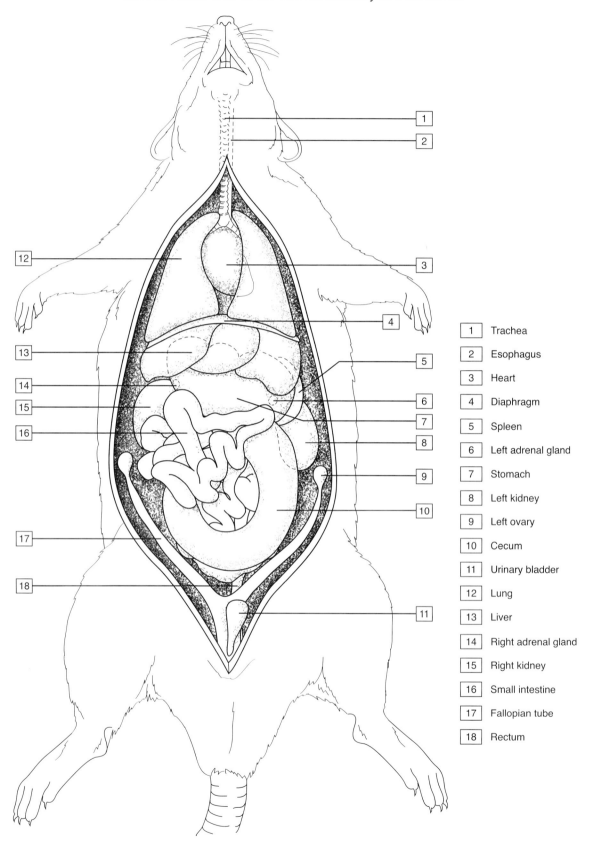

1	Trachea
2	Esophagus
3	Heart
4	Diaphragm
5	Spleen
6	Left adrenal gland
7	Stomach
8	Left kidney
9	Left ovary
10	Cecum
11	Urinary bladder
12	Lung
13	Liver
14	Right adrenal gland
15	Right kidney
16	Small intestine
17	Fallopian tube
18	Rectum

Saunders Veterinary Anatomy Coloring Book

FIGURE 8-12

Serpentine: ventral view of the internal anatomy of a snake

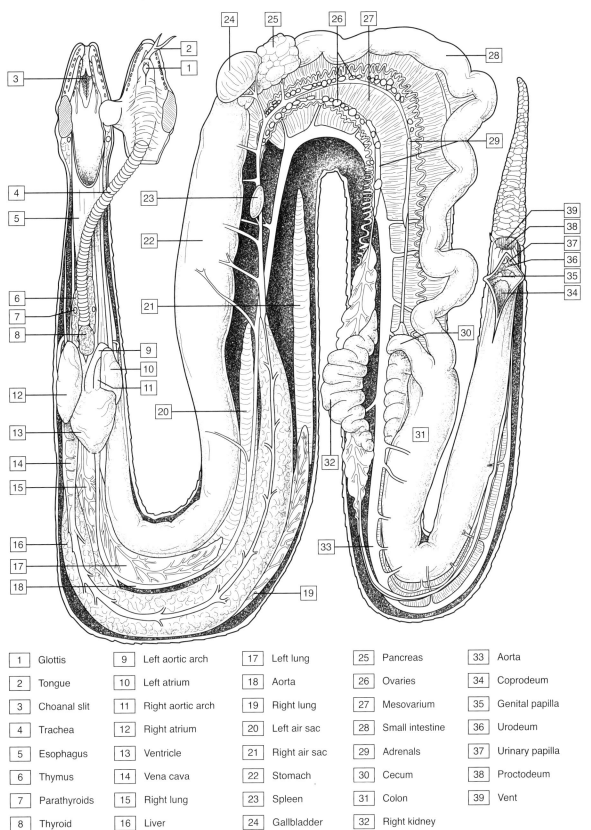

1	Glottis	9	Left aortic arch	17	Left lung	25	Pancreas	33	Aorta
2	Tongue	10	Left atrium	18	Aorta	26	Ovaries	34	Coprodeum
3	Choanal slit	11	Right aortic arch	19	Right lung	27	Mesovarium	35	Genital papilla
4	Trachea	12	Right atrium	20	Left air sac	28	Small intestine	36	Urodeum
5	Esophagus	13	Ventricle	21	Right air sac	29	Adrenals	37	Urinary papilla
6	Thymus	14	Vena cava	22	Stomach	30	Cecum	38	Proctodeum
7	Parathyroids	15	Right lung	23	Spleen	31	Colon	39	Vent
8	Thyroid	16	Liver	24	Gallbladder	32	Right kidney		

FIGURE 8-13

Serpentine: dorsal view of the heart of a snake

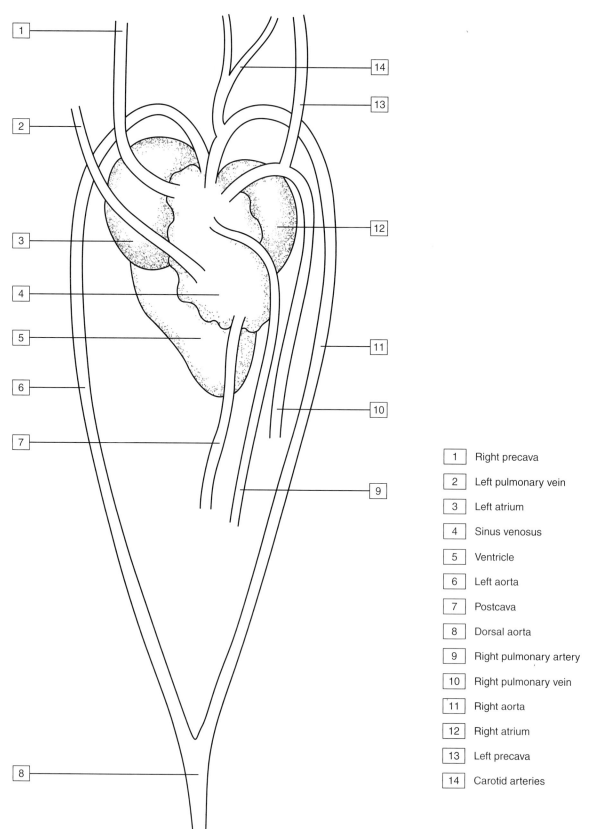

1	Right precava
2	Left pulmonary vein
3	Left atrium
4	Sinus venosus
5	Ventricle
6	Left aorta
7	Postcava
8	Dorsal aorta
9	Right pulmonary artery
10	Right pulmonary vein
11	Right aorta
12	Right atrium
13	Left precava
14	Carotid arteries

FIGURE 8-14

Lacertilian: ventral view of the internal anatomy of a Savannah monitor lizard

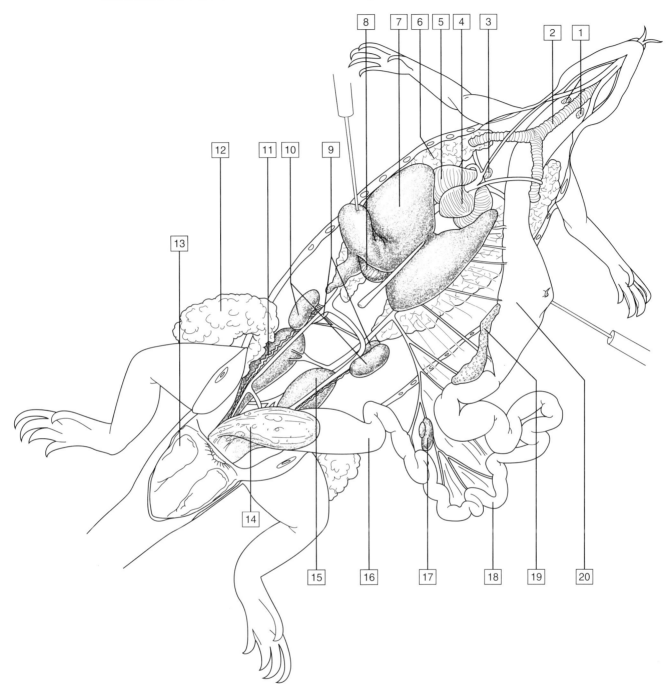

1	Parathyroids	6	Lung	11	Vas deferens	16	Colon
2	Trachea	7	Liver	12	Fat pad	17	Spleen
3	Thyroid	8	Gallbladder	13	Hemipenis sac	18	Small intestine
4	Ventricle	9	Adrenal glands	14	Bladder	19	Pancreas
5	Right atrium	10	Testes	15	Kidney	20	Stomach

FIGURE 8-15

Lacertilian: cloacal anatomy of a female lizard

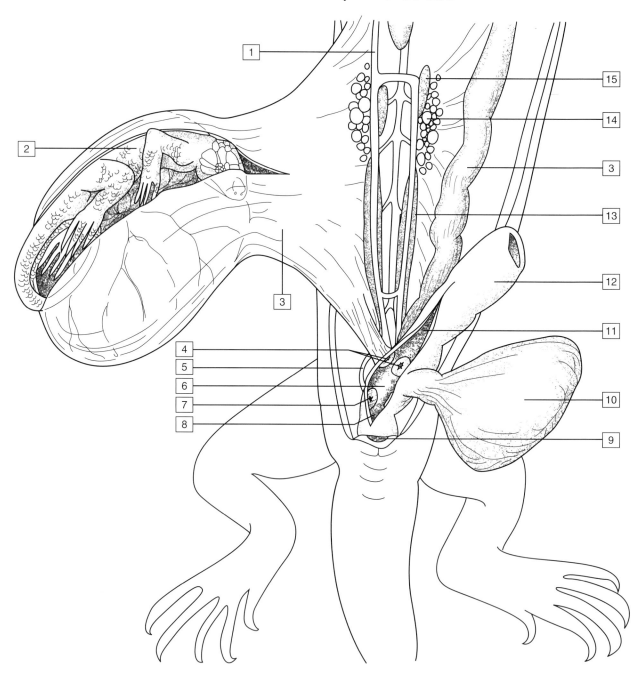

1	Vena cava	5	Ureter	9	Vent	13	Kidney
2	Near-term fetus	6	Urodeum	10	Urinary bladder	14	Ovary
3	Shell gland	7	Urinary pore	11	Coprodeum	15	Left adrenal gland
4	Genital pores	8	Proctodeum	12	Distal colon		

FIGURE 8-16

Chelonian: ventral view of the internal anatomy and
nomenclature of the plastron and carapace scutes of a tortoise

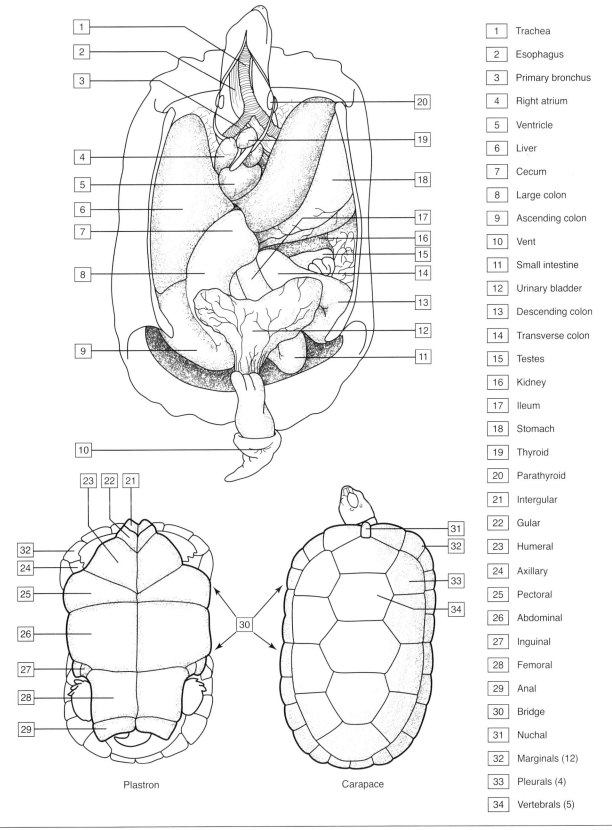

1	Trachea
2	Esophagus
3	Primary bronchus
4	Right atrium
5	Ventricle
6	Liver
7	Cecum
8	Large colon
9	Ascending colon
10	Vent
11	Small intestine
12	Urinary bladder
13	Descending colon
14	Transverse colon
15	Testes
16	Kidney
17	Ileum
18	Stomach
19	Thyroid
20	Parathyroid
21	Intergular
22	Gular
23	Humeral
24	Axillary
25	Pectoral
26	Abdominal
27	Inguinal
28	Femoral
29	Anal
30	Bridge
31	Nuchal
32	Marginals (12)
33	Pleurals (4)
34	Vertebrals (5)

Plastron

Carapace

FIGURE 8-17

Bufotenine: ventral aspect of the internal anatomy of a frog

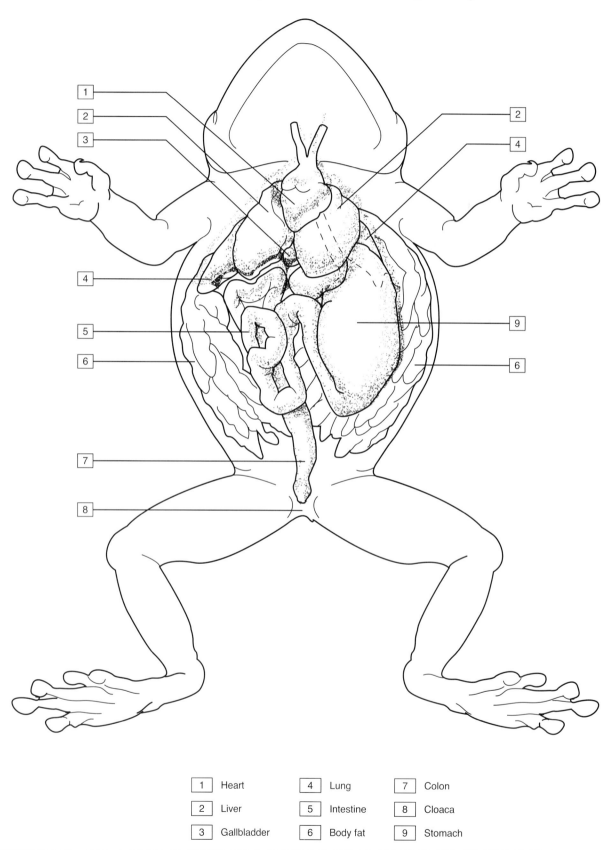

1	Heart	4	Lung	7	Colon
2	Liver	5	Intestine	8	Cloaca
3	Gallbladder	6	Body fat	9	Stomach

Saunders Veterinary Anatomy Coloring Book

FIGURE 8-18

General circulation in the noncrocodilian reptile

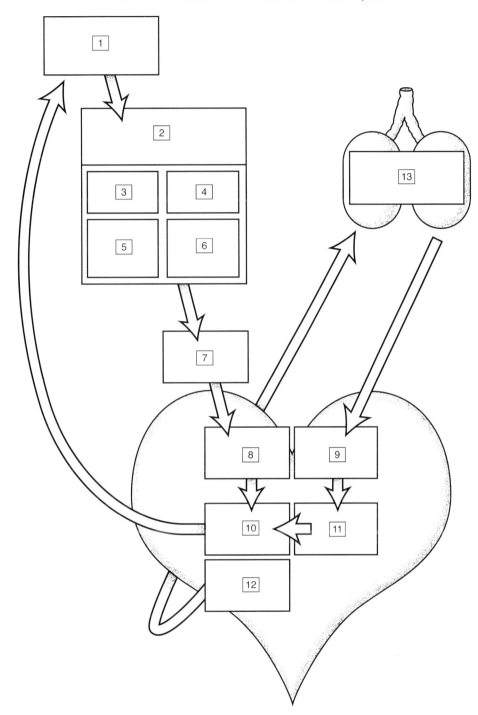

1	General circulation	5	Left hepatic vein	9	Left atrium	13	Pulmonary circulation
2	Major vessels returning to the heart	6	Post-cava	10	Cavum venosum	
3	Left precava	7	Sinus venosus	11	Cavum arteriosum	
4	Right precava	8	Right atrium	12	Cavum pulmonade	